Reviews By Students Of Shifu ___ ini

Shifu Michael K___ ___etime of experience in ___ ___ed quickly and use i___ ___seases. I highly recomme___ ___uld not be surprised if you re___ ___actice the qigong that you become one of Shifu's regular students.
Chuck Steg, Qigong Teacher & Daoist Priest

Shifu Michael offers us an uncomplicated description of ancient qigong exercises and theory for health and wellness in modern times. A wonderful way to discover our unique self-healing abilities whether it be for strength and balance, energy, stress reduction, and meditation.
Linda Anderson, Qigong Practitioner

This book is a treasure. As a long time student of Shifu Michael's Qigong and meditation classes, I can attest to the healing power of bringing these teachings into a regular practice that will truly enrich your life.
Terri Navé, Qigong Teacher

This book contains essential guides to various qigong techniques to help us maintain our health. Shifu Michael expertly explains step-by-step how we can have agency over our health with daily qigong practices, including forms specific to lung health. It's an essential book for people of all qigong knowledge levels.
Alyse Stuck, Qigong Student

An exceptionally valuable tool and asset for Qigong practitioners of any level. In these times, one certain thing is the importance of taking responsibility for our own mental and physical health. "Qigong for Humanity" gives us all the ability to do just that, fine-tuned for the challenges of our day and age.
J. Thatcher May, Qigong Student

I have studied with Shifu Michael for 10 years. His new Qigong book gives clear descriptions of class sessions and concisely describes targeted practice for lung and immunity support. He includes context information and clarification of profound Taoist knowledge to support a deep and healthful practice.
Dan Needham, Qigong Practitioner, and Daoist Initiate

This is a rare book – such a thorough and clear guide on Qigong routine is precious. This work is universal as it presents the practices that strengthen our general immune defenses. The guide is very practical in its hands-on clarity of description and reads like a personal conversation with the author who generously shares his knowledge, experiences, and ideas. Under the outward practicality of Shifu Michael's teachings, a thoughtful reader will find an abundance of deeper wisdom based on complex concepts of Chinese medicine and the Daoist worldview. The book is a wealth of condensed knowledge.
Svetlana Shklarov, MD, Ph.D., Qigong Student

Appreciations to my Qigong students,
practitioners, reviewers, proofreader, resources,
and family support and patience.

Books by Shifu Michael Rinaldini

A Daoist Practice Journal: Come Laugh With Me, 2013

A Daoist Practice Journal: Circle Walking, Qigong & Daoist Cultivation, 2016

A Daoist Practice Journal: Qigong, Seasonal Food Cures & Daoist Cultivation, 2019

A Daoist Grows In The Heart: Journals Of A Modern-Day Western Daoist Priest, 2020

Qigong

A Beginners To Advanced Guidebook

Shifu Michael Rinaldini (Li Chang Dao)

Qigong & Daoist Training Center
American Dragon Gate Lineage

Qigong, A Beginners To Advanced Guidebook
Copyright © 2020 Michael Rinaldini
All Rights Reserved.

ISBM: 9798649625678
Imprint: Independently Published

Disclaimer
The intention of this publication is for guidance and suggestion relevant to the subject matter presented. Readers should use their discretion and consult their doctors before engaging in any of the physical exercises. The author shall have neither liability nor responsibility to any person or entity concerning any loss or damage caused or alleged to be caused, directly or indirectly by reading or following the instructions in this book.

Credits
All illustrations of exercises and the Taiqi Ruler copyrighted by Michael Rinaldini © 2020
Cover photograph by Michael Rinaldini © 2020

Table of Contents

Introduction
Introduction to Book 10

Part 1
Chapter 1: Warm-Ups 16
Chapter 2: Purge & Tonify 22

Part 2
Chapter 3: Five Healing Sounds 31
Chapter 4: Seasonal Qigong 42

Part 3
Chapter 5: The Metal Element and the Immune System...... 58

Part 4
Chapter 6: The Theory Behind The Exercises 72

Part 5
Chapter 7: Daoist Meditation 103

Part 6
Chapter 8: The Future Of Qigong: Chong Mai Qigong 114

Part 7
Chapter 9: The Conclusion 121

Bibliography 129
About The Author 132

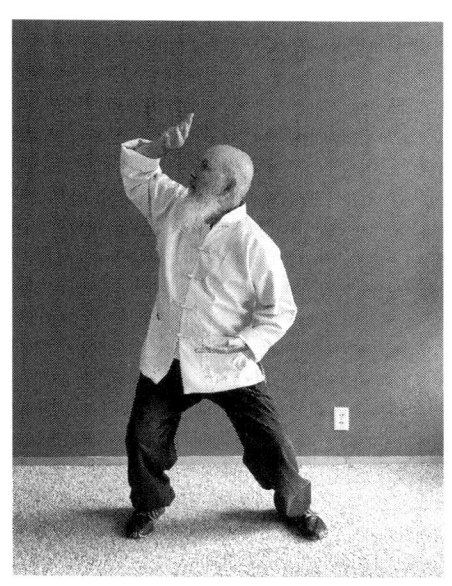

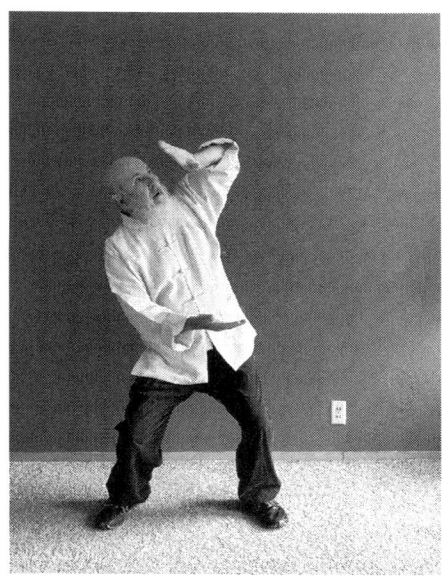

Wuji Palms Facing Heaven

Introduction

Introduction To Book

Qigong has been part of my life for the last 25 years. If you define Qigong in the broader sense of the word, it would include meditation, and that would make Qigong part of my life since my twenties. My involvement with Qigong would then be about 50 years.

As a whole, my Qigong practice has been integrated into my Daoist practice which is the way that Qigong and Daoism initially originated. So personally, these two paths have been with me for many, many years. Regarding my writings for the past 8-10 years, I have focused on a journal writing approach that has explored my Qigong and Daoist practices as they relate to my experiences as a modern-day western Daoist priest. Since 2013, I have written and published four books on these practices. As I was finishing my fourth book, back in late 2019, I decided to write a straightforward book on Qigong. I intended to start writing it during the 2020 summer. I had an idea of writing a book based on how I teach Qigong classes in Sebastopol, California. Additionally, I would provide more details about the exercises that I was presenting. For instance, I would first describe how to practice the Swimming Dragon exercise. Then, I would provide an analysis of the exercise explaining things like which meridians were being stimulated or strengthened. I would include Five Element considerations, and other relevant factors. And I would discuss the benefits for that specific exercise. That was my original intention, and I also intended to provide a concise introduction to Chinese Medicine. Not the kind of information that acupuncturists study, but the basic concepts like the meridians, the extraordinary vessels, the basic Five Elements (Metal, Fire, Water, Wood, and Earth). Also, the key concepts of Qigong cultivation like the Three Treasures (Jing, Qi, and Shen), the three Dantians, and the important concept of Wei Qi would be discussed. I would also provide a thorough explanation of the Qigong State which I talk about in class. I wanted to give my local students a thorough foundation in Qigong so when I mention any of these key teachings in class, they would have a firm understanding of them.

That was my plan, and still is but I decided to add a few other areas of concentration. The second area of concentration is a discussion of how to boost immunity. A weak immune system or what is referred to in Chinese medicine as the Wei Qi field is responsible for protecting the body from a host of illnesses. It is common in Chinese medicine to say that a strong Wei Qi field will protect you from the Rebellious Qi. Thus, I will include in this book a special section that deals with this subject.

The third area of concentration is for students who are ready to go beyond the basics. They will find areas of study like the advanced Qigong State, a specialized Qigong form called Chong Mai Qigong, and an advanced form of Daoist meditation called Zuowang.

Before moving forward with the Qigong exercises, allow me to present some basic definitions of Qigong and then some guidelines to keep in mind for practicing Qigong, regardless of the style or orientation.

What is Qigong?

First, what exactly is Qigong? In Chinese, the word "qigong" is broken down into two characters, "qi" and "gong." The "qi" is energy, life force and so many other variations on those meanings. My Qigong teacher, Master Wan Sujian refers to it as "Nature Qi." I frequently refer to it as the energy of the universe, the moving force behind all forms of creation. In short, I call it "Universe Qi."

Regarding the "gong" of Qigong, that is the skill of working with the Qi. When the Qigong practitioner has developed their skills through hard work, constant practice, trial, and error, and has arrived at the most effective way to use the Qi for the good of others and noble causes, then, you can say, he has perfected his/her "gong" of working with the "Qi." And yes, there is also a virtue in working with the Qi. After all, I didn't mention it earlier, but Qi is also referred to as "Universal Intelligence." Thus, to gain the skills of working with "Intelligence" one must possess virtue.

In conclusion, Qigong is the skill of working with the life force, the Qi. As a Certified Senior Qigong Teacher of the National Qigong Association (NQA), I would like to share with the reader, their definition of Qigong:

> What is Qigong? Qigong can be described as a mind-body-spirit practice that improves one's mental and physical health by integrating posture, movement, breathing technique, self-massage, sound, and focused intent. There are likely thousands of Qigong styles, schools, traditions, forms, and lineages, each with practical applications and different theories about Qi ("subtle breath" or "vital energy") and Gong ("skill cultivated through steady practice"). From NQA, nqa.org

Basics of Qigong

The practice of Qigong requires following basic guidelines that apply to most forms of Qigong unless a specific exercise requires a contrary procedure.

Below are some of the most common features of Qigong:

1. There is a feeling of standing tall as if you are being pulled up to the heavens, and at the same time, you feel you are being pulled down to the earth.
2. The tip of the tongue is either touching the palate behind the upper teeth, or the tip of the tongue is extending straight up touching the roof of the mouth.
3. The shoulders, upper back, and chest are all relaxed.
4. Breathing in through the nose using the basic deep abdominal breathing method. Exhaling through the mouth is common though.
5. Generally speaking, the movements are slow and done in a relaxed manner.
6. The number of repetitions varies according to the exercise. There is no benefit to being obsessive about repetitions.
7. When the exercises are done in the Qigong State, the benefits are greatly amplified.

You are now ready to attend class. Oh, I should mention that there is another Qigong basic, and that is silence and stillness. Sometimes, students ask me how old is Qigong, and what is the most essential aspect of Qigong? The original primitive forms of Qigong are ageless, just like the origins of Daoism. And Qigong has its roots in Daoism. If I were to say what is the most powerful aspect of Qigong, I would say, it is the power of silence and stillness. Silence and stillness are energy, or more accurately said, silence/stillness equals Qi. (Silence/Stillness = Qi) From this equation arises the conclusion, if silence/stillness is Qi, and Qi is Universal Life Force, then silence/stillness is the most powerful source of healing. So, to bring this realization back to ordinary Qigong practice, I say, every time you practice Qigong, even the most basic warm-ups, practice in the state of silence and stillness. My local students are very familiar with my pronouncement when we do Qigong Circle Walking. I say, "Take your stillness for a walk." When you practice Qigong like this, you have moved from a beginner to a more advanced student.

Now, you are ready to begin your Qigong class. And please do so in the true spirit of feeling like you are in an actual class. You should also feel free to vary your class workouts. It is an underlying Qigong principle to not perform the same Qigong routine all the time. In the Wuji Palms Facing Heaven exercise portrayed on page eight, I am performing one of my favorite Qigong exercises. This exercise is perfected when there is the greatest variety of movement. In conclusion, use this book to develop a solid introduction to Qigong, but allow yourself to go deeper into the mysteries of Qigong.

Part 1

Chapter 1: The Warm-up Exercises

Twisting and Turning the Upper Back #1
While turning from side-side, the hands tap the back of the neck and the mid-back.

Twisting and Turning and Looking Back #2
As you continue turning side-side, your hands tap the outer hips as you look to see the back of your heels. Allow the hips to move.

Up and Down Bending Forward #3
Bend forward to the ground with your hands, and slightly tilt backward when you straighten up.

Theory & Benefits
These three movements are the beginning of loosening the whole body, but especially the spine. I learned them from two Chinese medical and Qigong doctors who run a spine clinic in China. The function is to open and stretch the vertebrae of the spine to allow a harmonious flow of Qi through the meridians and vessels of the back. The main meridian on the back is the Bladder meridian.

Loosening The Joints Of The body

Head-Neck
Turn the head, side-side. Next, look up and down. Next, roll the head around, both directions.

Theory & Benefits
The main physical benefit is to loosen up the vertebrae and muscles of the neck by moving in all directions. This will relieve any stiff neck problems and over time will restore flexibility to the neck. Keeping the neck flexible and relaxed supports the smooth flow of Qi which moves up and down the neck passageways through several meridians and vessels: Bladder, Large Intestine, Stomach, Governing and Conception Vessels

Shoulders
Roll the arms around in a big circle, then, roll the shoulders around.

Hips
Make big circles with hips, both directions.

Small Circles
Make small circles with the pelvic bones, i.e., visualize the tip of the tailbone moving in small circles, both directions. Next, tilt the tailbone forward, and backward.

Bend Side-Side
With your hands on your hips, slightly bend to both sides.

Knees
Sink, hands on knees, and make circles, both directions. Next, hands on knees, make outward circles, both directions, then, inward circles.

Ankles
Rotate each ankle, make full circles, both directions, and toes up and down.

Theory & Benefits
The shoulders, hips, knees, and ankles are all benefited similarly to the spine and neck. Loosening the joints of the entire body has the positive effect of opening and stimulating the smooth flow of Qi to the whole body. All the meridians and vessels are equally benefited by allowing the joints to move easily without discomfit or pain, and thus supporting optimum Qi flow.

Meridian tapping
Stretch upwards, then, bend down to the ground. Straighten up, tap the lower back or Mingmen area, with a soft fist or open palm.

Tap down the back of the legs, up the inside of the legs, down the outside of the legs, up and down, several times. Firm tapping.

Tap the chest, all around, out to the shoulders but below the collar-bone, up and down along the sternum.

Tap down the inside of the arms to the open palm, and then, turn the palm downward, and tap up the arms to the shoulder, and even base of the neck. Repeat, down, and up the arms several times.

Tap back of head, tap forehead, and tap all around the head. Press firmly along the eyebrows, press with fingertips along the ridge above the eyes, and the ridge below the eyes.

Theory & Benefits
Tapping the pathway of the twelve meridians opens and stimulates the energies of the entire body including the extraordinary vessels which are located along the same pathways as the twelve meridians. The exceptions to this rule are the Governing and Conception Vessels. However, when you tap the whole body even these two vessels are included in the tapping. Tapping the meridians is also a method of supporting and nourishing the Five Elements: Fire, Earth, Metal, Water, and Wood. The Mingmen point is along the Governing Vessel, at the level of the navel.

The Mingmen point is of great importance in Qigong and human health, so I will present additional information on it now. It is located on the spine between the second and third lumbar vertebrae, across from the navel. It is related to the

Kidney energy system, which is the powerhouse of the body providing extra energy to any organ. Whenever there is a Qigong exercise that directly or indirectly affects the Mingmen, special consideration should be given to that exercise.

Furthermore, the Mingmen is of importance because it is considered the sum of the two kidneys, meaning, it is both Yin and Yang – water and fire. That is why you frequently see references to the Mingmen point as the Mingmen Yang Fire. In summary, when the Mingmen is strong there is a great benefit derived from practicing Qigong.

Dragon Looks Behind
This is a whole-body twist and turning side-side, while one hand reaches above as if pushing out, the opposite hand drops to the side as if pushing to the ground. (Figure 1) As you turn side-side, you are looking over your shoulder. Even your head is turning to look back, including your eyes. The opposite heel rises slightly in the direction you are turning.

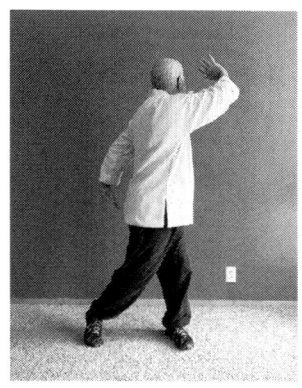

Figure 1

Theory & Benefits
This is a relaxing movement for the whole body. Sometimes I practice it on its own just to loosen up and feel good. It is also a concluding exercise to the warm-ups ensuring that the body is loose and flexible and prepared for the deeper work of purification and tonification.

You are now finished with the warm-ups.

Chapter 2: Purge & Tonify

The Basic Taiji Ruler
The next exercise is a preliminary cleansing or detoxing. In my practice, we have a simple technique called, The Basic Taiji Ruler. If you do not have a Taiji Ruler, imagine holding a wooden stick in your hands. The stick is about a foot (10.5 in.) in length and has a round sphere in the middle of it. (Figure 2)

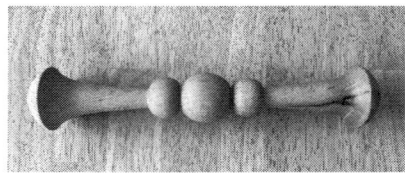

Figure 2

Because this exercise has many steps to it, I will only be presenting a simplified version of it.

Preparation. Stand with your feet in your normal shoulder-width posture. Hold the ruler (or imaginary ruler) just below the navel. Breathe into the Lower Dantian, feel the belly expand and contract. Allow your thinking mind to sink into this place. Feel surrounded by healing energy, especially from above.

Exercise
Reach your hands/ruler up and pivot towards your right. The left leg is slightly bent, and the right leg is

straight but on a steep angle. Exhale as your hands move down your leg to the foot, while saying the healing "shuu" sound. (See the Five Healing Sounds section) (Figure 3)

Every time you finish the downward movement, reach up, inhale, and feel as if you are gathering and absorbing fresh Universe Qi from above. Repeat many times. (Figure 4)

Continue on the right side, first, reach up, pivot to the center, take a couple of breaths, pivot to left, and repeat on the left side. Finish on the left side, pivot to the center, lower the ruler to the navel.

Closing. Stand still, breathe deep into the Lower Dantian. Feel refreshed, cleansed. Extend the feeling of breathing to the whole body. Practice a few minutes.

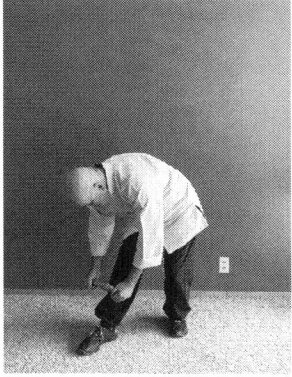 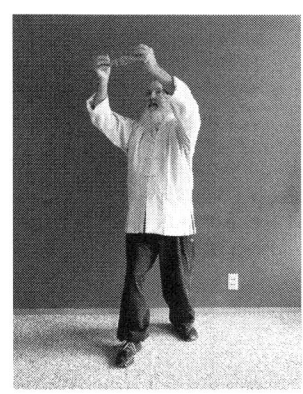

Figure 3   Figure 4

Theory & Benefits
The Basic Taiji Ruler is practiced immediately after the warm-ups and before the main Qigong forms because it serves the function of cleansing and detoxifying the body. I always repeat the following words in class as we begin: "let go and release your tensions, stresses, and anything else that is bothering you." We use our intentions and willpower to detach from any negative energy or what is referred to in Chinese Medicine as "evil influences" or "rebellious Qi." We are also gathering Universe Qi when we reach up and imagine healing energy descending on us. We imagine it going deep into our Three Dantians, replenishing the meridians and vessels, and helping to push out any impurities. We quietly pronounce the healing Liver sound as we release and let go, shuu.

Swimming Dragon
The Swimming Dragon Qigong involves turning the upper body to each side. Pay attention to the details of the technique to get the maximum benefits.

Preparation. Stand with your feet far apart, as in the traditional horse stance-the feet are wider apart than the shoulders, and the knees are slightly bent. This preparation position is crucial and will affect the correct performance of this Qigong. The hands move side-side in a specific pattern. The hands move at the same pace, though, one hand faces upward, and the other hand faces downward. This form could easily be called Heaven and Earth Palms.

Exercise

Start. Inhale as your left-hand moves across the front, palm facing up. As the left-hand moves across the front, the upper body is turning to the right side. The left hand completes its movement by touching the right shoulder (Figure 5), and then, exhaling the hand sinks to the side, palm faces downward, as the body turns to the right side. The right arm fully extends to the back.

At the same time, the right hand has begun moving to the left, the palm facing up, and touching the left shoulder. (Figure 6) The two hands and arms are in sync when one hand touches the opposite shoulder, and the other arm is fully extended to the back. At that point, the back palm faces up, and the movement repeats itself. Practice for a minimum of five minutes.

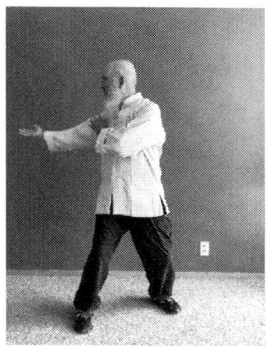
Figure 5

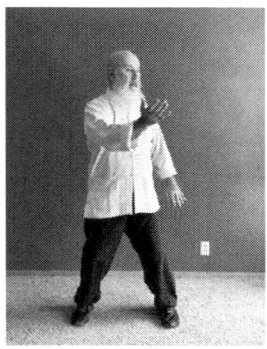
Figure 6

25

Theory & Benefits
Swimming Dragon is a powerful Qigong exercise. It benefits the whole external body on a physical level by stretching the muscles, tendons, and ligaments. It opens, stimulates and strengthens all the meridians and vessels due to the whole body twisting to the rear as much as possible. And internally, the organs, especially the liver, gallbladder, stomach, spleen, and pancreas are all compressed and then relaxed. This compression and relaxation acts to squeeze out blood from those organs, and then allows a fresh supply of blood to return to them. Swimming Dragon acts on the entire body from the head and neck down to the ankles and feet. When performed correctly, you feel that your feet have worked their way out of your shoes. That indicates the full-twisting and turning of swimming like a dragon. The main benefits are for the Middle Burner consisting of the organ systems mentioned above.

Open and Close
After finishing Swimming Dragon, transition directly to Open and Close.

Preparation. Stand with your feet shoulder-width apart, hold the hands at waist level, palms facing each other.

Exercise
Inhale and separate your hands, exhale and close your hands, this is Open and Close.

Open and Close is usually the starting practice for getting into the Qigong State. Relax and breathe as you perform these simple movements.

Theory & Benefits
Open & Close is one of the simplest Qigong exercises but its function, application, and roots are deep in the practice of Qigong. I learned from my Chinese Qigong teachers that this method of gathering the Universe Qi is commonly practiced by the sick and dying in China. They do this when all else has failed and the only thing the person can do for themselves is this simple movement. There are many stories of recovered health from this exercise alone.
The theory behind Open & Close is straightforward Qi & Gong. That is, we benefit from the work or skill of using the Universal Qi. Additionally, when we perform this exercise we go through a transformation process that is called, entering the Qigong State. This state is a profound experience that is an essential component of what makes Qigong, Qigong. See the section on the Qigong State for a full discussion on it.

Wan Sujian's Three Dantian Tonifying
This Qigong form tonifies the three Dantians: Upper, Middle, and Lower. This is a simple version of gathering Universe Qi into the three Dantians.

Preparation. Stand with the feet shoulder-width apart for a few relaxing moments.

Exercise

Raise the hands above the head, palms facing each other, inhale as you expand your hands to the sides. Exhale as the hands come in close to the top of the head. (Figure 7) Feel that you are pulling in Universe Qi and directing it to flow into the Upper Dantian. Perform this exercise for a couple of minutes.

Next, lower your hands to sides, and exhale while the hands sink, (Figure 8) inhale straighten up, raising the hands. Feel that you are absorbing Universe Qi and directing it to flow into the Middle Dantian. Repeat. Practice this for a few minutes.

Next, bend the upper body towards the feet, and open and close the hands, like in Open and Close. (Figure 9) Feel that you are pulling Earth Qi up from deep in the ground, and directing the Qi to flow up the leg meridians (Kidney, Spleen, and Liver) to the Lower Dantian. Repeat. Practice this for a few minutes.

Finish by standing up, and reaching the hands up as if deep into the sky. Pull the hands down slowly and place them on the Lower Dantian. Feel the Universe Qi gathering deep in the Lower Dantian, and going into storage in the Kidneys.

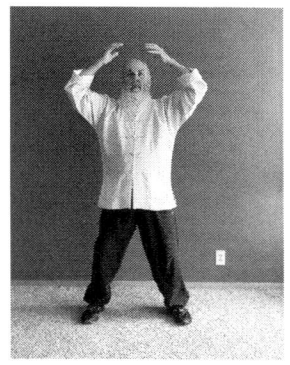 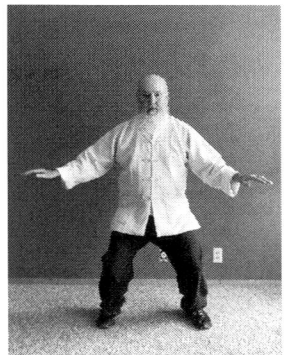

Figure 7   Figure 8

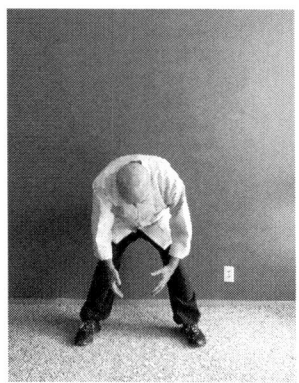

Figure 9

Theory & Benefits
Master Wan Sujian is my main Chinese Qigong teacher who lives in Beijing, China. During my four visits to his center, I learned his Qigong routine called BaguaHundunGong. In addition to his Three Dantian tonifying exercise, I also learned from him the Basic Taiji Ruler and circle walking. The purpose of the Three Dantian

Tonifying exercise is to gather Universe Qi into the Dantians: Upper, Middle, and Lower. The Dantians are explained in more detail in the Chinese Medicine section. When we tonify the Dantians, we are also strengthening the whole body through the meridians and vessels which are linked to the entire energy system of the body. Sometimes this energy system is called the Matrix of the body, mind, and spirit.

The other important consideration for this form is to pay extra attention to breathing into the Mingmen area when bending towards the ground (Figure 9). Feel the low back area expand and contract as you breathe. Visualize Universe Qi flowing deep into this area vitalizing your Kidney Qi, Lower Dantian, and ultimately nourishing the Three Treasures of Jing, Qi, and Shen. Some teachers and ancient sources say the Mingmen point needs to open first before any other points along the Governing and Conception Vessels.

Part 2

Chapter 3: The Five Healing Sounds

The second half of our Qigong class will include a variety of exercises. The choice of exercises will depend on several factors: personal preference by myself, the teacher, or requests by the students or a particular health issue dominant in the population.

The Five Healing Sounds

A good place to start is with the universal Qigong exercises known as the Five Healing Sounds and the seasons of the year. There are many variations of the healing sounds. They are all equally valid, the following sounds are what I learned many years ago. An easy way to learn the healing sounds is to practice them in association with the Five Elements and the seasons.

Wood/Spring
A quick review of the Wood/Spring season, according to Chinese Medicine and Five Element Theory shows that the Spring is associated with the Wood Element and the Liver and Gallbladder organ/meridians.

The healing sound for the Wood Element and the Liver is "shuu." It sounds just like the word, shoe, but the sound is drawn out as you are exhaling.

Theory & Benefits
The healing sound for the Wood Element produces a special quality of kindness, generosity, and forgiveness. It helps to dissipate the heavy emotions like anger, frustrations, and depression. When the Wood energy is flowing smoothly, it is said the Liver is "free and easy wandering."

In my experience, healing sounds are the most powerful when aligned with physical action. The most basic action is a lightly pressing circular massage over the area of the liver.

Clenching The Fists
Another basic movement is blending the "shuu" sound with one of the Eight Brocades Qigong called Clenching The Fists. It is a punching movement to the front or the sides while standing in the wide-horse stance. Starting with clenched fists at your side, one hand at a time punches. It is best done outdoors where you can see trees, grasses, bushes, anything of a wood nature. You imagine punching into the green natural elements and pulling back into you the healing green energies. This benefits your Liver and Gallbladder organs/meridians. Practice as long as you wish.

Theory & Benefits
Clenching The Fists is one of the historical Eight Brocades or Baduanjin Qigong. It originated with a semi-legendary Chinese military officer, General Yue Fei, who developed a form of Qigong which was broken down into eight separate exercises. According to legend, he taught his soldiers these exercises to help them maintain physical fitness during a military campaign.

Fire/Summer
A review of the Fire/Summer season, according to Chinese Medicine and Five Element Theory is that the Summer is associated with the Fire Element and the four organ/meridians of the Heart, Small Intestines, Pericardium, and Triple Warmer. (See below for the special healing sound for the Triple Warmer)

The healing sound for the Fire Element and the associated organs is "haa." It is a soothing sound coming from deep in the chest. Massage your hands over your heart area while making the calming relaxing sound of "haa."

Theory & Benefits
The healing sound for the Fire Element produces a feeling of joy and gladness for life. It enhances your ability to express your love to others and culminates with gratitude of love for the world.

Rolling The Ball
A simple Qigong exercise for blending the "haa" sound and the related Heart, Small Intestines, Pericardium, and Triple Warmer meridians of the arms is the Rolling The Ball Qigong exercise.

Exercise
Rolling The Ball is a simple rolling or circulating movement of the arms. You are moving your arms in a complete circle, and the only special condition is that the palms are constantly facing each other as if you are holding a giant ball. (Figure 10)

Then, every few minutes, you step forward with one leg, and both hands push forward as you exhale with the "haa" sound. See the healing Qi flowing to the Heart. Do a few pushes, and then return to the rolling the ball. Repeat the same pushing a few minutes later with the other leg.

The only thing I have not mentioned is that while you are rolling the ball, you can be walking around in small circles in a relaxed but yet energetic state.

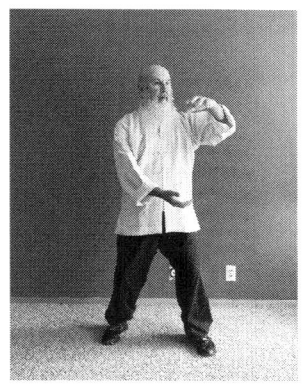

Figure 10

Theory & Benefits
Rolling The Ball stimulates all the Fire meridians of the arms: Heart, Small Intestine, Pericardium, and Triple Warmer. This exercise is particularly beneficial in the summer to regulate and cool the Fire organs.

The Triple Warmer meridian is the only meridian which is not directly related to an organ system. It is sometimes called the "San Jiao" and is considered mysterious energy. The Triple Warmer has its healing sound of "Heeeeee."

Theory & Benefits
This sound benefits the balancing of fire and water in the body. It also produces a sense of calmness, smooth flowing Qi, and balance. It regulates the three regions of the body: Upper (heart, lungs); Middle (liver, spleen, stomach); and Lower (kidneys, bladder, intestines).

Earth/Late Summer
A review of the Earth/Late Summer season, according to Chinese Medicine and Five Element Theory is that the Late Summer is associated with the Earth Element and the Spleen and Stomach organ/meridians.

The healing sound for the Earth Element and the associated organs is "whoo" It is a soft sound coming from deep in the throat.

Theory & Benefits
The healing sound for the Earth Element produces a mental sense of balance and equanimity, and you will worry less. You will also have a greater sense of fairness, openness, and rootedness.

Massage your hands over your Spleen area or, over the Stomach which is directly below the sternum while making the "whoo" sound. If you experience frequent belching, heartburn, or reflux it is recommended to massage the Stomach area, but emphasizing a downward direction.

Small Turning The Belt Vessel
A Qigong exercise for blending the "whoo" sound with the Spleen meridian is the Small Turning The Belt Vessel.

Exercise
In Small Turning The Belt Vessel exercise, you make a small circle with your palms facing down. The hands are held close to each other and your body sways side-side following the circular movement of the hands.

Your mind imagines a warm current of energy flowing around the waist at the level of the navel and the Mingmen.

After a while, move your hands in the reverse direction.
Breathe in and out normally with the movements, and on the exhale make the healing "whoo" sound and imagine healing Qi flowing to the Spleen and Stomach.

Theory & Benefits
The Belt Vessel is the only extraordinary vessel that circulates the waist. It connects the navel and the Mingmen in its path around the waist. It benefits the Middle Burner and all the internal organs, from the liver to the spleen. It is also beneficial for the kidney energy as it directly passes through the Mingmen and related Bladder meridian on the lower back.

Metal/Fall
According to Chinese Medicine and Five Element Theory, the Fall is associated with the Metal Element and the Lungs and Large Intestines organ/meridians.

The healing sound for the Metal Element and the Lung and Large Intestines is the "Sssssss" sound. It sounds like a hissing sound made by placing the tongue behind the upper front teeth and blowing. The upper and lower teeth are gently touching each other. Sometimes it is described as the hissing sound of air escaping a tire tube.

Massage your hands over your Lung areas, either on the chest or on the upper back while making the purifying hissing sound. Sometimes, I gently tap the chest while hissing.

There are many Qigong exercises for blending the hissing sound with Qigong breathing exercises which are very beneficial for the Lungs. (I will include these exercises in a separate section on the Lungs)

Theory & Benefits
The healing sound for the Metal Element produces a strong immune system and supports the mental qualities of righteousness, justice, and an inner strength against grief and sorrow.

Water/Winter

The last healing sound we will practice is part of the Water Element and Winter season. According to Chinese Medicine and Five Element Theory, this is the Element and season to focus on the Kidneys and the Bladder organs and meridians.

The healing sound for the Kidneys is "chruee." It is the only healing sound that is two syllables. First, a short "chru" that almost sounds like a "tree" sound. It is followed by a longer "ree" sound, much like the "haa" or "whoo" sounds. Thus we get a "chru-ree" sound. Sometimes, you may see this sound spelled "Chui."

Theory & Benefits
The healing sound for Water Element produces a sense of courageous, powerful willpower, and a deep sense of interconnectedness. It also fosters our inner state of stillness and serenity.

Do the same type of massage that you did for the other sounds, but this time focus on the Kidneys on the back. However, because of the difficulty of reaching the Kidney areas on the back, I usually reach as far to the back as possible and gently tap with soft fists that area.

A simple but powerful exercise to blend the "chruee" sound with the Kidney energy is called Hold The Feet.

Hold The Feet
Preparation. Stand with the feet shoulder-width apart and hands over the navel area. Place your attention on the Mingmen area and visualize a strong Kidney fire at that location.

Exercise
Inhale and raise the hands, keeping the attention on the Mingmen Yang Fire. (Figure 11) Exhale and simultaneously bend the body until the hands grasp the feet or back of ankles. (Figure 12) while visualizing the Kidney Yang Fire energy sinking (along the Bladder meridian) to the bottom of the feet (Kd 1). At the same time, you are making the healing "chruee" sound.

Feel powerful Kidney and Water Element energy going deep into the Lower Dantian and Kidneys. Repeat this process several times and perform a closing by standing still and imaging Kidney Qi going into storage in the Lower Dantian and Kidneys.

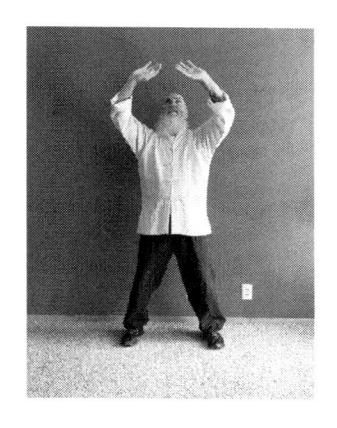

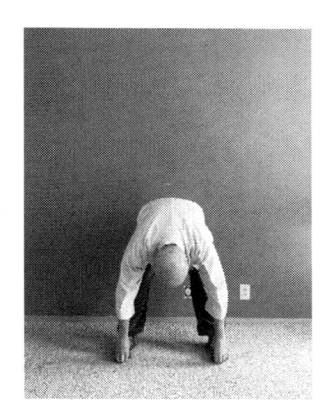

Figure 11   Figure 12

Theory & Benefits
Hold The Feet stimulates the Kidney and Bladder meridians. It warms the Mingmen Yang Fire of the lower back. This exercise is particularly beneficial in the winter to warm the internal organs. Focus on the stream of warm energy sinking to the feet and eventually to Kd 1 on the front third of the bottom of the feet. In addition to that visualization, imagine a powerful beam of light shooting straight from Kd 1 to the brain. This happens in an instant, so no use thinking about it, as it is actually pre-thinking. The theory behind this is that Kidney energy supports the brain.

Chapter 4: Seasonal Qigong

In your class workout, the exercises in this section will normally follow the warm-ups, the Basic Taiji Ruler, and the Master Wan's tonifying exercises. The choice of exercises for the second half of the class will depend on several factors. One factor that I consider for every class is Seasonal Qigong. Let's start with a couple of exercises for the summer and winter.

Seasonal Qigong for the Summer and Winter

Five Animal Frolics

We will start with two exercises from the popular Qigong form called the Five Animal Frolics. The practice of the frolics can follow the seasons of the year. The main frolics that I practice are the crane for the summer and the bear for the winter seasons.

Bear and Crane Frolics
The Five Animal Frolics are a major Qigong exercise. In the summer (and autumn) you can practice the Crane Frolic. And in the winter, it is beneficial to practice the Bear Frolic. Here is the technique for the Crane Frolic.

Crane Frolic
Preparation. Stand in the usual shoulder-width posture for a few relaxing moments. The hands are

placed at chest level with the fingertips touching and the palms facing up.

Mental Preparation. Feel like you are the crane. Think of being the crane as you softly breathe: your bones are light, porous, though strong; your feathers are white which protects you from the heat of the sun. You are very calm and patient and you feel deep inside you a loving peacefulness.

Exercise
Inhale as the hands raise a few inches and exhale as they sink a few inches.

Next, raise your hands along your sides, palms facing down, but only half-way up, and down, half-wing flying. Inhale up, exhale down. (Figure 13) The hands are soft and gently flex during this movement. An alternative is to form the fingers into the cranes' beak by holding the fingertips touching as they move up, and relax as they move down. (Figure 14)

In the next step, the hands reach above the head with the back of the hands facing each other but do not touch, full-wing flying. (Figure 15) Same breathing, inhale up and exhale down. Breathe deep into the Lower Dantian and also the chest. This is relaxed breathing. No forcing the chest to expand or excessively expanding the belly. Feel free to use the crane hand posture.

You can practice both of these movements, the half-wing flying, or the full wing flying for as long as you want. The next movement is optional as it requires great leg strength and balance.

Simply put, you take turns shifting your weight to one leg at a time, and raising the other foot. The foot can be raised a few inches or up to opposite the knee of the other leg. As you do this, the arms are doing the half-wing flying, and your body is moving up and down gracefully. Again, same breathing pattern, inhale up and exhale down. Sometimes, it helps to maintain balance if you keep your eyes open and stare at the floor about 6 feet in front of you.

Practice with both legs equally, and if you are constantly struggling with your balance, decrease the height of raising your foot, or leave your big toe on the ground as the heel raises.

Closing. Return to your preparation posture with the hands at chest level and perform a minute of the up and down movements. Finish with the palms of your hands placed on the Lower Dantian. Feel refreshed and revitalized. Feel the Universal Qi absorbing deep into the Lower Dantian and the Heart and Lungs.

The Crane Frolic can be added to the routine for strengthening the lungs and boosting immunity.

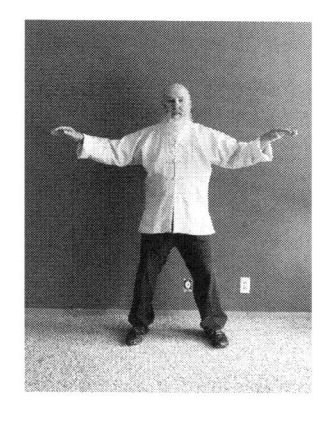

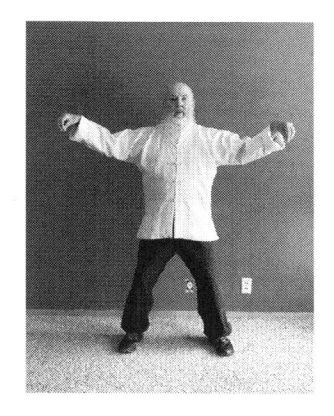

Figure 13   Figure 14

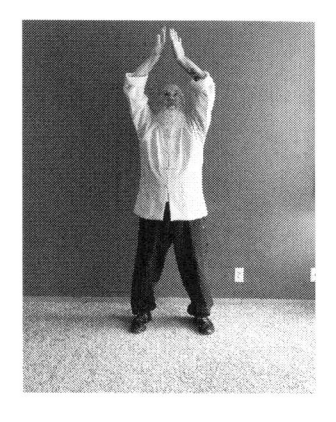

Figure 15

Bear Frolic
Preparation. Stand in a wide stance, feet further apart than shoulder width. The knees are bent and the degree of how much bent depends on the overall strength of your legs. Your weight is on both legs equally. The following description is a modified

version to easily allow you to learn the basics of the Bear Frolic.

Mental Preparation. Feel you are a big, powerful grizzly bear. You weigh 700 lbs. and your bones are extremely strong. You are rooted in your stance and the earth.

Exercise
Breathing. You exhale whenever you turn to the sides, and inhale when you return to the center or front.

While standing, raise your hands, elbows bent, above your shoulders, as if holding a huge tree branch. Imagine you are standing in front of your mountain cave and are moving the tree branch away from your cave.

Step 1: Bear Turns To Side
Turn your upper body 15 degrees to the side without moving the hips or legs. Feel the strength of your legs and lower back. Return to the center, and then to the other side. Remember the correct breathing mentioned above. Practice about 5-10 times, return to the center, and lower the arms. Hands-on navel. Brief rest. (Figure 16)

Step 2: Bear Pushes To The Side.
Return to starting position of raised hands. Lower the hands to the front of the chest, slightly to the side, in

the position of pushing an object. The palms are bent back at the wrists.

Similar to the turning of step 1, and push both hands to the side. Return hands to center, and push both hands to the other side. Alternate back and forth feeling like you are pushing the tree branch away from the cave. Practice about 5-10 times, return to the center, and lower the arms. Hands-on navel. Brief rest. (Figure 17)

Step 3: Bear Pushes To The Ground
Return to starting position, push both hands to the side, (Figure 17), then bend at the waist, allowing the hands to complete a smooth downward swing and over to the other leg.

Slowly pull up the hands along the leg and upper body, about 1-2 inches from the chest, until you are standing straight again. Push the hands out to the side and follow the same pattern to the other side. Alternate back and forth, feeling like you pushed the tree branch away and now you are rolling it away from the cave. Return to center, rest hands on the navel. (Figure 17-19)

Throughout each of these three movements, concentrate your mind on your lower back, Lower Dantian, and Mingmen.

Closing. Return to center with the hands-on navel. Feel that you stimulated Universal Qi to circulate throughout your body, especially through the Kidney and Bladder meridians. Feel the Qi absorbing deep into the Lower Dantian and the Kidneys.

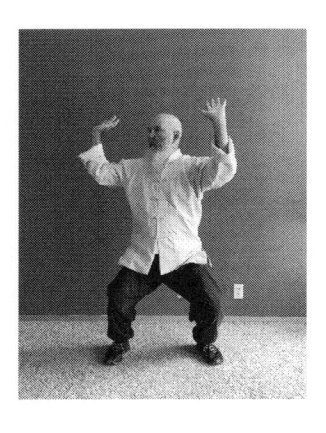

Figure 16

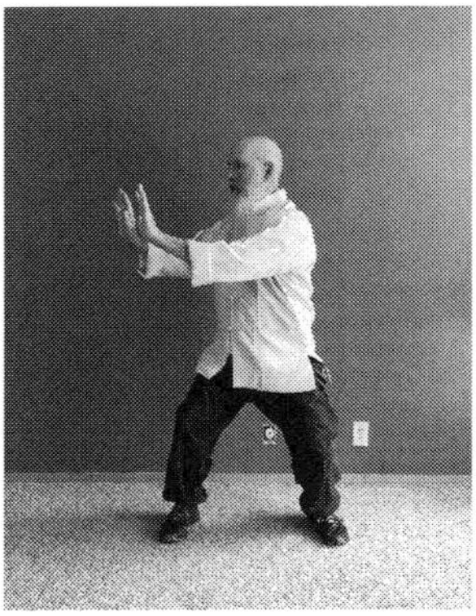

Figure 17

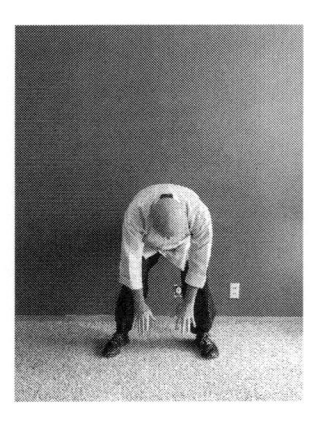

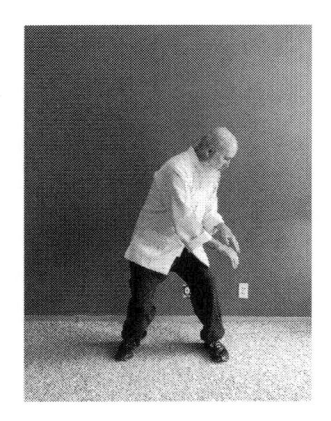

Figure 18

Figure 19

Theory & Benefit
The Five Animal Frolics is the oldest Qigong system still practiced today. It was created by Hua Tuo (A.D. 110-207) who is considered the Father of Chinese Medicine. The system consists of five forms modeled after five animals: bear, crane, tiger, deer, and monkey. Overall, the frolics strengthen the internal organs and the external muscles and other tissue. All the meridians and vessels are benefited, with each frolic having specific benefits. The crane benefits the Fire and Metal Element and the bear benefits the Water Element.

Seasonal Qigong for the Autumn

Drawing The Bow
This exercise is one of the Eight Brocades Qigong which has numerous versions. In my classes, I emphasize that this exercise can be used to tonify all the organ/meridians. And yet, Drawing The Bow can be used to strengthen any individual organ/meridian. The factor which determines the purpose of the exercise is the intention of the mind. In other words, if I want to focus on the Kidneys, for instance, I would emphasize the sinking of the body and the turning of the waist to the side. If I want to focus on the Heart or Lung channels, I would emphasize the extending and contracting movements of the arms as well as the breathing. And so on and so on. For our purpose now, we will practice Drawing The Bow as a way to strengthen the Lungs.

Preparation. Stand in the horse-stance with the knees bent. Breathing is in the Lower Dantian and it is deep, soft, and smooth. The preparation position for the arms is one hand in front of the right side of the chest and the other hand half stretched out to the left side. The left elbow is bent and the index and middle fingers of the left hand are extended while the other fingers are grasped together.
Exercise

Version 1
Inhale and then exhale as you slowly extend the left arm outward to the side. At the same time, the right hand is pulling back holding a soft fist. Imagine you are drawing the bow.

Inhale and smoothly shift the arms to the other side. Exhale, and repeat the same movement towards the right side of the body. Repeat many times, both sides of the body. (Figure 20)

Version 2
Same preparation and movements as version 1, except for the breathing.

Inhale as you extend one arm and pull back with the soft fist. Feel the full breathing in the Lower Dantian and the chest.

Exhale as the arms shift smoothly to the other side, and inhale extending and pulling back as previously done on the other side. Repeat many times, both sides. (Figure 21)

Closing. Return the hands to the Lower Dantian and feel that you have tonified the Lungs.

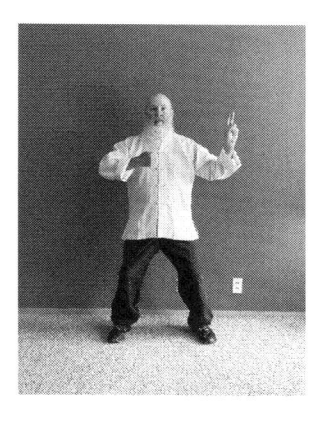

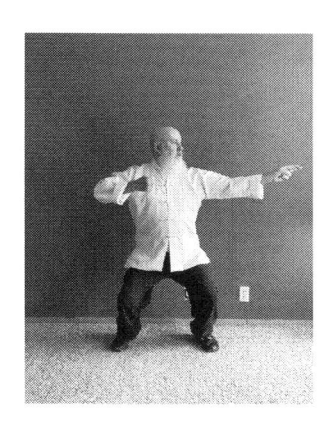

Figure 20   Figure 21

Theory & Benefits
This exercise is good for all the meridians and also for specific meridians based on one's intentions. It is also good for the muscles and sinews of the arms and upper torso. A general guideline in all the Eight Brocades is to perform them smoothly and avoid jerky movements. In class, I frequently remind students to do the exercises as if you were in slow-motion.

Seasonal Qigong for the Late Summer

Double Hands Hold Up The Heavens
Single Hands Push To Heaven And Earth.

Both of these exercises come from the Eight Brocades Qigong just like Clenching The Fist and Drawing The Bow. In my classes, I emphasize Double Hands and Single Hands to tonify the Triple Warmer meridian which indirectly benefits the Earth Element and the Spleen and Stomach organ/meridians.

Double Hands Hold Up The Heavens
Preparation. Stand with feet shoulder-width apart and arms relaxed at the sides.

Exercise
Inhale and raise your arms above your head with the palms facing up and the fingertips pointing toward each other. Fully extend the arms. The hands need to be flexed backward.

Closing. Exhale and lower the arms to the sides. The whole body feels relaxed. Repeat many times. (Figure 22)

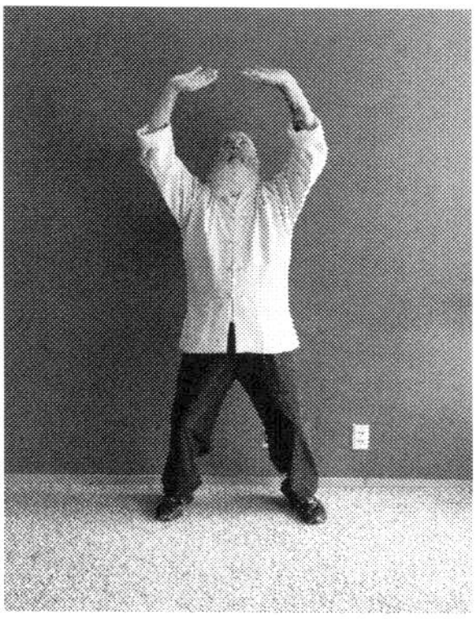

Figure 22 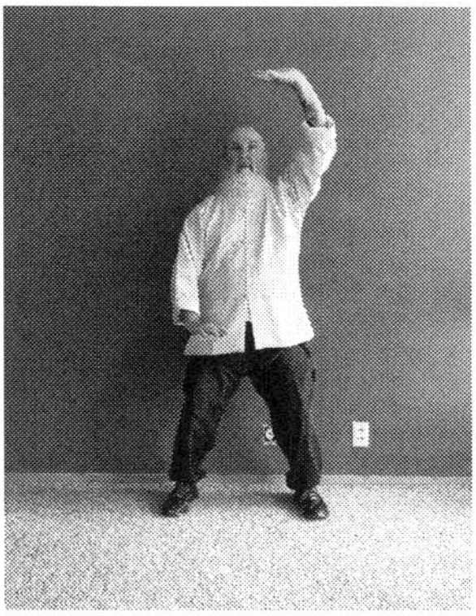   Figure 23

Single Hands Push To Heaven And Earth
This exercise also stimulates the Triple Warmer meridian and the Spleen and Stomach. This exercise is very similar to Double Hands Hold Up The Heavens, except that the hands move in opposite directions.

Preparation. Same preparation as Double Hands Hold Up The Heavens.

Exercise
Inhale and raise the left arm, palm facing up, and push the right hand down along the side. Fully extend the arms. The hands are flexed back and you have a sensation of pushing opposite directions. The hands need to be flexed backward.
Exhale and the hands come back to the center in front of your abdomen and you immediately inhale alternating the other hands pushing up and down.

53

Closing. Exhale and lower the arms to the sides. The whole body feels relaxed. Repeat many times. (Figure 23)

Theory & Benefits
These two Eight Brocades exercises stimulate the Triple Warmer, meaning they benefit the three levels of the body: upper, middle, and lower areas. The Double Palms may have more of an effect on strengthening the lungs, and the Single Palms may have a greater effect on the spleen and the stomach. You are flexing the hands the correct amount if you feel a slight tingling sensation in the wrist. Eventually, this tingling sensation will go away if you perform this movement or similar flexing movements regularly.

Seasonal Qigong for the Spring

Dragon Chases The Pearl
This exercise stimulates the movement of the Liver Qi by encouraging a strong flow of Qi up the Governing Vessel (the back) and down the Conception Vessel (the front). The turning and moving up and down action encourages the Liver Qi to become "free and easy wandering."

Preparation. Stand in a slightly wider shoulder-width stance. Hold your hands in the front of your body as if you are holding a ball. Imagine this is a ball of fiery energy that the Daoists call the Pearl of Immortality.

Exercise
Inhale and turn to your right with your hands reaching towards the base of the spine. (Figure 24) Continue inhaling and moving the hands up the back, over the head. (Figure 25) Exhale as the hands move down the front of the body towards the Lower Dantian.

Repeat, turning to the left side, reaching up, over top of the head, and back to Lower Dantian. (Figure 26) Continue this movement many times, moving energy up and down the Governing and Conception Vessels.

Closing. Bring hands back to the Lower Dantian, feel that you have stimulated the movement of Qi throughout the body but especially the Liver Qi.

There are many other Qigong exercises for the Spring and Wood Element. One of them, I already mentioned, and that is the Basic Taiji Ruler. During the Spring, Seasonal Qigong focusses on cleansing and purging exercises. The Basic Taiji Ruler is ideal for this purifying action.

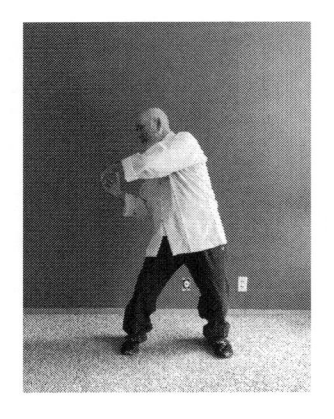

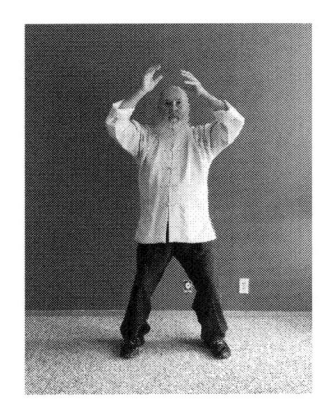

Figure 24   Figure 25

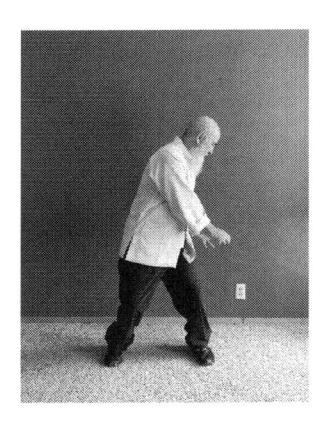

Figure 26

Theory & Benefits
The Wood Element and the Liver energy need to flow smoothly as the saying goes: free and easy wandering. That is also the name of a famous patent Chinese herbal formula: Free and Easy Wanderer. If we do not allow our emotions to flow freely, we are creating blockages for ourselves,

which eventually become the root of diseases in the body, mind, and spirit. Dragon Chases The Pearl encourages fluid movement of Qi up and down the Governing and Conception Vessels which supports the openness of the Liver and Gallbladder meridians.

Part 3

Chapter 5: The Metal Element, the Immune System, and Wei Qi

Section 1: Introduction

This section focuses on keeping our Lungs, immune system, and Wei Qi field strong. There are many common, ordinary ways of doing this. Some practical suggestions are, first of all, to maintain a regular Qigong practice. But also, to eat healthy according to the seasons. We can take extra vitamin or herbal supplements. We can go on more frequent walks or other inside or outside exercises and get plenty of rest. What all of these practices are doing is giving us a strong immune system. In Chinese Medicine and Qigong theory, the western notion of the immune system is correlated to the energetics of the Metal Element and the Lungs. This system also includes the skin as the skin is considered the external lungs. The other component of the energetic body that needs consideration is called the Wei Qi. The Wei Qi is described in the section on the basics of Chinese Medicine. So for now, you can say, to keep ourselves strong against any invading negative influences we have to maintain a high level of breathing capacity and vitality, and a strong protective shield of Wei Qi.

The following outline and description of exercises is a sample of exercises I shared with my local Qigong students. The understanding behind this Five Element plan is to strengthen the Lung Qi. The theory states that if you want to strengthen the Lung Qi or Metal Element, you also support the nourisher or mother element, which is the Earth Element and the related organs and meridians (Spleen and Stomach). And since the Metal Element is the parent of the Water Element and related Kidney and Bladder organs and meridians, it is important to keep those energy systems strong so they do not become burdens on the parent-the Metal Element. The Lung Qi would also be supported directly as well.

In summary, if the Lung Qi is the focus, you would also support the Spleen Qi and the Kidney Qi. However, when you read the section on the Wei Qi, you will see that there is reason to believe that the Spleen Qi is just as important, and maybe more important than the Lung Qi. (Part 4 explains the Five Element system in great detail.)

Section 2: Exercises To Boost The Health Of The Lungs, Immune System, and Wei Qi

Spleen – Lung – Kidney Immune Boosting

Spleen

Swimming Dragon - The twisting of the waist stimulates the organs-kidneys, spleen, liver. (Figures 5-6)

Bear Frolic - Slow, ponderous, very strong movements warm the body and strengthen the Spleen Qi. (Figures 16-19)

Five Element Organ massage - Spleen massage: yellow color, "whoo" inhale trust, openness, and sincerity and exhale self-doubt, obsessiveness, and worry.

Food Cures For Keeping The Spleen Healthy
In addition to Qigong, the Spleen is greatly nourished by diet. In general, the first step to take is to eat a diet of cooked foods that have a warming energy nature. The next step is to avoid cold and damp foods like ice cream and other high sugar content foods. This includes junk foods of all kinds, cold soft drinks, raw vegetables, and even ice-cold water. Below are some food recommendations from my book, *A Daoist Practice Journal: Qigong, Seasonal Food Cures & Daoist Cultivation.*

Dr. McCann says, "eating cold foods burdens the Spleen and Stomach, and this is more damaging during the Yin and colder times of the year when the body is trying to consolidate its Yang warmth" (2017, 27).

Astragalus (Huang Qi) for immunity and Spleen Qi, and Dioscorea (Shan Yao) for tonifying the Spleen Qi.

I like Dr. McCann's first recommendation to combat the heat and dampness of summer. These environmental influences have a depressing effect on the Spleen energy. "In Chinese medicine, the Spleen is susceptible to dampness, the disease evil associated with the Earth phase. The Spleen governs the flesh and the four limbs. Damp evils encumber the flesh of the four limbs making them feel heavy and weary" (2018, 25). And what is the thing to do according to McCann, take an afternoon nap. Napping will give you a boost when it is hot and damp outside, and it'll assist your Spleen vitality.

Along with this emphasis on gathering and storing the strong Yang Qi deep inside, we need to keep up the discipline of eating wisely. By this, I mean to not give in to your cravings for sugary and cold foods, like refreshing cold sodas and ice cream desserts. The dampness contained within these foods and drinks will seriously weaken the Spleen energy, which will have a detrimental influence on your digestion. Instead of these outcomes, it is better to clear heat and dampness by eating fresh summer salads, emphasizing cucumbers, raw tomatoes, and the melons.

Specific foods good for the spleen: oats, brown rice, most vegetables, lean meats/poultry, potatoes, sweet potatoes, beans, ginger, garlic, onion family, rice congee, peanuts, cherries, peaches, and more. Meals prepared as stews or in crockpots are especially nourishing for the spleen and digestion.

Lungs

Dragon Looks Behind - Stretches Lung and Large Intestine meridians of the arms. (Figure 1)

Five Element Organ massage - Lung-chest massage and tapping, visualizing white light purifying the lungs. Sssssss sound – hissing like a snake.

Drawing The Bow - Stretches and opens the Lung and Large Intestine arm meridians and opens the chest cavity. (Figures 20-21)

Crane Frolic - Develops balance, lightness, endurance, agility, and stillness. It releases the spine and relaxes the whole body. It strengthens the heart and lungs by increasing the circulation of Qi in the upper body. (Figures 13-15)

Kidney and Lung Breathing - Bend forward, hands hanging in Open and Close, and breathe Qi into your Mingmen/kidneys. Straighten up, hands-on lower back area, slightly lean backward and breathe Qi into your chest/lungs. (Figures 27-28)

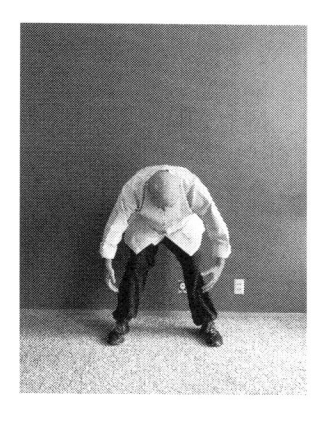

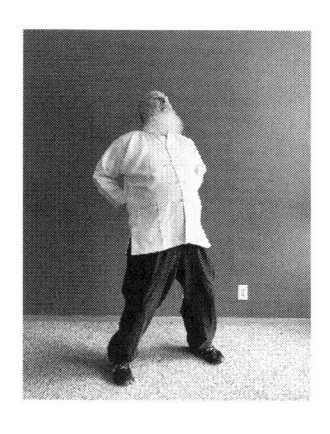

Figure 27   Figure 28

Peter Deadman Breathing - Slowly raise arms in front, palms face each other, continue to expand outward. Being careful to not over-expand the arms. Breathing: One long, slow inhale into the Lower Dantian for the full movement. Exhale as the arms come back to the front and sink. Imagine the Lower Dantian filling up with Universe Qi. Visualize the Qi going deep into the lungs. (Figures 29-30)

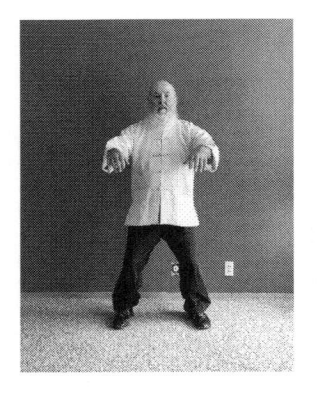

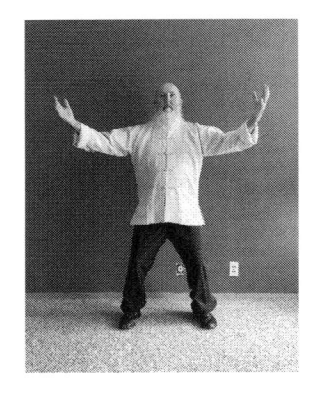

Figure 29　　　　　　　Figure 30

Metal White Energy Cloud – Imagine being surrounded by a cloud of white healing Qi. Practice the basic Qigong exercise of Push-Pull. Exhale, turning to the side and push out toxins from the right lung. Inhale, pull in healing white energy to the right lung. Turn to the other side and perform the same Push-Pull, releasing toxins, absorbing healing Qi to the left lung. Alternate back and forth. (Figures 31-32)

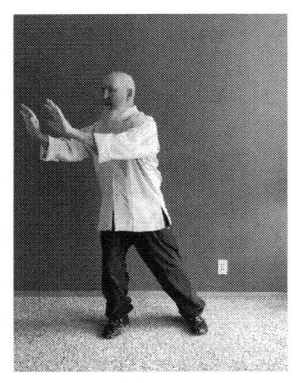

Figure 31　　　　　　　Figure 32

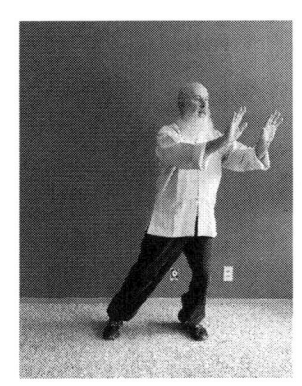

Ken Cohen Crane Breathing - It is all about breathing deep in the belly. The essence of the exercise is slow breathing as you slightly bend backward and then forwards while standing and concentrating on the breath coming and going from the abdominal region, the Lower Dantian. You can also practice this exercise while sitting straight in a chair. Also, place the palms over the navel area, and when you lean forward, press the abdominal area slightly. (Credit: Ken Cohen, *Qi Journal* Spring 2020) (Figures 33-34)

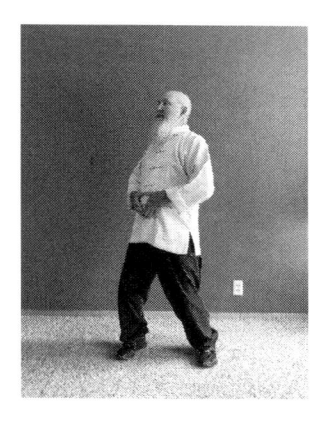

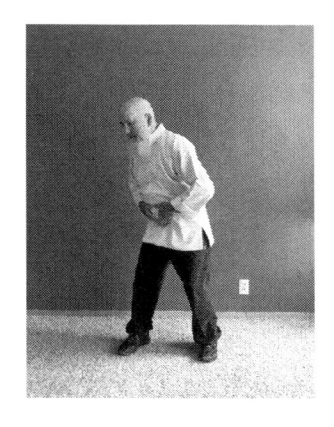

Figure 33   Figure 34

Kidney

Bear Frolic - Slow, ponderous, very strong movements warm the body and strengthen the Kidney energy, and builds vitality and great leg strength. (Figure 16-19)

Five Element Organ Massage – Massage or tap the kidneys in the back. Visualize blue/black colors, chruee sound. Inhale self-confidence, courage, and wisdom and exhale fear and loneliness.

Drawing The Bow - Strengthen Kidneys and waist by squatting down to firm your root as you draw the bow. Tucking in your tailbone emphasizes the Kidney area. (Figures 20-21)

Hold The Feet - Holding the feet strengthens the Kidney Qi, the waist, and the muscles/tendons and bones. Increased Kidney strength increases defenses against colds and other deficiency problems. Simple lean forward to the ground, hands holding the feet or behind the ankles. Imagine strong Kidney energy arising in the Mingmen and Lower Dantian. (Figures 11-12)

Moon Yin Tonifying
This Qigong is intended to tonify the whole body with the Yin energies of the moon. It is best practiced on a clear night when the moon is either full or close to being full. And since it involves bending backward, the best time of the evening is when the moon is not straight above.

Preparation. Stand in a relaxed stance facing the moon. Place your hands on your Lower Dantian.

Breathe deep in the belly for a minute with your eyes closed.

Exercise
Inhale (open eyes) and slightly bend back looking directly at the moon. Feel like you are inhaling the universal Yin energies of Nature. Direct the energy to flow into your body passing through the nose, lungs, and filling the Lower Dantian. Exhaling bending forward a little and releasing any toxins of the body. (Feel free to use the healing "shuu" sound on the exhale)

Closing. Practice as long as you want and then return to standing still and feel the Yin energy going deep into the Kidneys for storage.

Summary Of Exercises To Benefit The Spleen, Lungs, Kidneys, and Wei Qi Field

In most of the above exercises, visualize that you are practicing in a white healing cloud. See this white cloud as especially healing for the Lungs and Spleen and wrap this healing cloud around your whole body. This is your Wei Qi, that is, your energetic immune system, protecting you on all levels but especially from external pathogens.

Section 3:

Brief reports on strengthening the Immune System

1. A study was circulated on Facebook about a research project that showed the benefits of exercise and keeping the immune system strong. Its main premise was that regular exercise may reduce the risk of acute respiratory distress syndrome (ARDS).

   A review by Zhen Yan, Ph.D., of the University of Virginia School of Medicine, showed that medical research findings "strongly support" the possibility that exercise can significantly increase immune system functions. Research findings discovered an endogenous antioxidant enzyme.

   Powerful Antioxidant
   Yan, the director of the Center for Skeletal Muscle Research at UVA's Robert M. Berne Cardiovascular Research Center, compiled an in-depth review of existing medical research, including his own, looking at an antioxidant known as "extracellular superoxide dismutase" (EcSOD). This potent antioxidant hunts down harmful free radicals, protecting our tissues and helping to prevent disease. Our muscles naturally make EcSOD, secreting it into the

circulation to allow binding to other vital organs, but its production is enhanced by cardiovascular exercise.

A decrease in the antioxidant is seen in several diseases, including acute lung disease, ischemic heart disease, and kidney failure, Yan's review shows. Lab research in mice suggests that blocking its production worsens heart problems while increasing it has a beneficial effect. A decrease in EcSOD is also associated with chronic conditions such as osteoarthritis.

Research suggests that even a single session of exercise increases the production of the antioxidant, prompting Yan to urge people to find ways to exercise. "Regular exercise has far more health benefits than we know.

"We often say that exercise is medicine. EcSOD set a perfect example that we can learn from the biological process of exercise to advance medicine," Yan said. "While we strive to learn more about the mysteries about the superb benefits of regular exercise, we do not have to wait until we know everything."

2. The following brief newsletter excerpt shows the relationship between the Lungs and Wei Qi.

   Below is an excerpt from a newsletter that I received on April 22, 2020. The source is Mayway Herbs (Mayway.com). They are a distributor of Chinese herbs for professional Chinese Medicine practitioners and are located in Oakland, California.

   The etiology of Wei Qi deficiency are manifold and determined by comprehensive differential diagnosis. The most common causes of deficient Wei Qi include Lung, Spleen, and Kidney deficiency patterns.

   The Lung governs the surface of the body, spreading proper movement of the Wei Qi to regulate opening and closing of the pores, and ensuring the healthy flow of Qi and blood to the skin's surface. When the Wei Qi is insufficient, the pores do not close correctly, and the skin is not sufficiently warmed and consolidated. The body's surface can then become vulnerable to the penetration of external environmental pathogenic influences.

From the above analysis, it is clear that if Qigong is going to be beneficial for boosting immunity it must tonify the lungs, spleen, kidneys, and the powerful Wei Qi protective field around the body.

Part 4

Chapter 6: The Theory Behind The Exercises

Basic Principles of Chinese Medicine
This section is a basic introduction to Chinese Medicine with a focus on the key principles of Five Elements, the Twelve Meridians and Eight Extraordinary Vessels, the Dantians, the Three Treasures of Jing, Qi, and Shen, and the concept of the Wei Qi.

The Five Elements

The Five Elements and their associations.
The Five Element theory is explanatory and emphasizes one-to-one correspondences, describing clinical processes and relationships to conceptualize the appropriate treatment.

The Five Elements are not elements in the regular sense of the term, but rather activities based on the observation of the natural cycles and interrelationships in both our environment and within ourselves.

All things in the universe and nature are inter-related. In an attempt to understand this inter-relationship the ancient Chinese developed a system known as the Five Elements. This system, when applied to mankind's health included the major organs, yin and yang, body tissues and fluids, senses, emotions, directions, colors, and the seasons of the year.

The five elements and related meridian/organ systems:
- Wood: liver and gall bladder
- Fire: heart, pericardium, triple warmer, and small intestine
- Earth: spleen and stomach
- Metal: lung and large intestine, and
- Water: kidney and bladder.

Within the Five Element theory, there are two main relationships or ways in which the elements interact.

Elemental Cycles

The first of these is the generating, nourishing (mother-child) cycle. This cycle describes how each element/phase serves as a mother, promoting the growth and development of the following child element/phase.

The controlling (grandparent-grandchild) cycle provides for a check and balance system among all of the elements. Within this cycle Earth, for example, provides a control for Water and is controlled by Wood.

The diagram below contains the nourishing and controlling cycles.

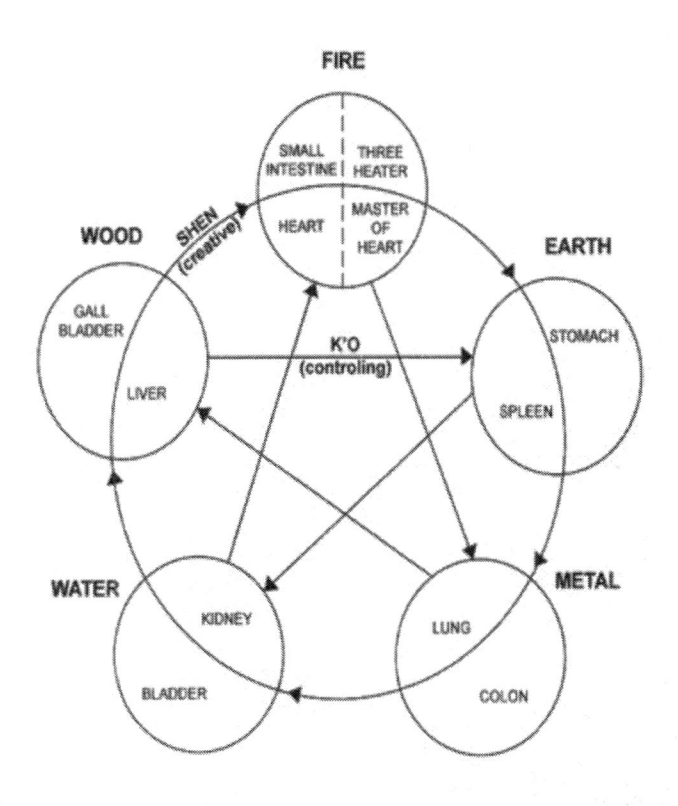

The Five Elements/Phases in a chart format:

	FIRE	EARTH	METAL	WATER	WOOD
Yin Organs	Heart & Pericardium	Spleen	Lungs	Kidneys	Liver
Yang Organs	Small Intestine & Triple Heater	Stomach	Large Intestine	Urinary Bladder	Gall Bladder
Sense Organs	Tongue	Mouth	Nose	Ears	Eyes
Tissues	Vessels	Muscles	Skin	Bone	Tendons
Tastes	Bitter	Sweet	Pungent	Salty	Sour
Colors	red	yellow	white	Blue Black	green
Sounds	Haa	Whoo	Sssssss	Chru-eee	Shuu
Emotion Sounds	Laughing	Singing	Crying	Groaning	Shouting
Odor	scorched	fragrant	rotten	putrid	rancid
Emotion	Love, joy, respect	Fairness, openness	Uprightness, courage	Gentleness	Kindness
Negative Emotion	Hate, impatience	Worry, anxiety	Sadness, depression	Fear	Anger

75

The Meridians or Channels

Narrowly speaking, one might say that the channels/meridians are 'spaces' in the body. In a larger sense, the concept of channel refers not only to the spaces but to everything wrapped within them. In this definition, the concept broadens to include not only the spaces within the connective tissues but also the structures and fluids held and brought together by these connective tissues. A channel is then like a river in that it includes the riverbanks and also the complexity of life within the water itself held by these banks. In the body, the channels are the groupings of connective tissue, that bring together the blood vessels, bones, lymphatic vessels, nerves, tissues, and interstitial fluids within their purview (scope). (Bisio 2012, 35)

More on the meridians.
The meridians are an invisible network of pathways, which transport qi throughout the body and particularly to the 12 major organs. These meridians are arranged in pairs or partners, one yin, which flows up the body, and one yang, which flows down the body (the traditional Chinese anatomical position is with the arms raised). Each pair is also connected at the extremities of the body so that where one ends the other begins.

The Lung Meridian is yin and is responsible for the absorption of heavenly Qi from the air and begins just below the collarbone and travels up the arm to the thumb.

The Large Intestine Meridian is yang and is responsible for elimination. It begins at the tip of the index finger and ends just below the nose.

The Spleen Meridian is yin and is responsible for moving and transforming food and distributing its energy throughout the body. It begins at the big toe and travels up the body to the side of the chest.

The Stomach Meridian is yang and begins just below the center of the eye and travels down to the side of the second toe, it is called the "sea of nourishment".

The Heart Meridian is yin and is known as "the root of life" and governs the "shen" or spirit. It begins at the armpit and travels up the arm to the little finger.

The Small Intestine meridian is yang and is responsible for "sorting of the pure and impure" of food and also emotions and philosophical concepts. It begins at the little finger and finishes at the side of the mouth.

The Pericardium Meridian is yin and is traditionally associated with the circulation of blood and the protection of the heart. It begins in the middle of the nipple and flows up the arm to the tip of the middle finger.

The Triple Warmer Meridian is yang and governs basic drives and appetite balance. It begins at the tip of the ring finger and ends at the tip of the eyebrow.

The Kidney Meridian is yin and stores energy for the entire body. It begins at the sole and travels up the leg and the side of the body to end just under the collarbone.

The Bladder Meridian is the most yang of all the meridians, it begins at the inner eye, runs over the head, down the back and legs, and ends at the little toe. This meridian is associated with fluid balance and energy like its partner the kidney meridian.

The Liver Meridian is yin and is responsible for good spirits and a sense of well-being. It begins at the big toe and ends between the 6th and 7th ribs.

The Gall Bladder Meridian is yang and is one of the longest meridians, beginning just below the middle of the eyebrow and ending at the tip of the fourth toe. It is very important for breaking down toxins and therefore promoting a more balanced state.

Below is a link to an extensive web page on the meridians and extraordinary vessels. Use them as references to visually understand the locations of the meridians/vessels and key points.

http://www.acumedico.com/meridians.htm

The Eight Extraordinary Vessels

The Eight Extraordinary Vessels regulate and influence the 12 meridians of the body. They store, distribute, and regulate the Jing and Qi throughout the body. Above, it was stated that the meridians are like rivers. Here, a useful image is that The extraordinary vessels are like lakes, which store a greater volume of water than the rivers.

The Eight Extraordinary Vessels are:

Conception Vessel (Ren Mai)
Governing Vessel (Du Mai)
Penetrating Vessel (Chong Mai)
Girdle Vessel (Dai Mai)
Yin linking vessel (Yin Wei Mai)
Yang linking vessel (Yang Wei Mai)
Yin Heel Vessel (Yin Qiao Mai)
Yang Heel Vessel (Yang Qiao Mai)

The Three Treasures of Jing, Qi, and Shen

The Three Treasures; pinyin: *sānbǎo* are theoretical cornerstones in traditional Chinese medicine and Daoist cultivation. They are also known as Jing, Qi, and Shen. They are three of the main notions shared by Daoism and Chinese culture alike. In the long-established Chinese traditions, the "Three Treasures" are the essential energies sustaining human life:

- *Jing* 精 "nutritive essence, essence; refined, perfected; extract; spirit, sperm, seed"
- *Qi* 氣 "vitality, energy, force; air, vapor; breath; spirit, vigor; attitude"
- *Shen* 神 "spirit; soul, mind; god, deity; supernatural being"

Thus begins the discussion of the three essentials of Chinese medicine and Daoist spirituality. These introductory explanations come from an initial internet-Google search. Consider these definitions as the most basic meanings and you should understand that there is a huge body of knowledge on these concepts. Thus, there are also contradictory ideas on many of these concepts.

Most literature on the Three Treasures limits their discussions to what is called the Post-Heaven material realm. This is the realm we are born into, live our lives, and then die. I think it is fair to say, that most Chinese Medicine focuses solely on this level. I include Qigong and Taiji into this generalization. My main reference to this understanding comes from the writings of Master Wu Jyh Cherng in his book, *Daoist Meditation: The Purification of the Heart Method of Meditation and Discourses on Sitting and Forgetting (Zuowang lun) by Sima Chengzhen. (*About Master Wu Jyh Cherng: (1958-2004), was a Daoist High Priest and Master of Meditation Rites and Ceremonies. Born in Taiwan and moved to Brazil in 1973. He was ordained into the Orthodox Unitary Order. He translated several Daoist texts, including the Zuowang lun mentioned above.)

To begin, The Three Treasures can be divided into two categories or realms. The first realm is Pre-Heaven, Pre-Existence, or what Master Wu Jyh Cherng calls Anterior Heaven. This is life before birth or existence when the Three Treasures are in a state of absolute unity. You can think of them as being in a state of stillness. This may also be called the state of Wuji, Emptiness, or Nothingness. Something makes them move out of this state of stillness, perhaps the energy of the Taiji primordial energy. The movement propels them to differentiate into the realm of Post Heaven or Existence. Now they are the three concepts or energies of life, which we are familiar with.

When we discuss the purpose of Qigong or Taiji, we come to a basic understanding that the purpose of these practices is to cultivate our Three Treasures to return them, or us, to the state from which they came, Stillness, or Pre-Heaven realm. And that's not easy.

Moving on, there are basics of these three treasures which we should have a good understanding.

Jing.
Jing is frequently called an essence. Often it is described as a sexual fluid, but it is more. Jing is not a physical substance, but it is rather close to the physical. It is a form of gross energy.

This Jing is our basic building block of life. The quality of life depends on the richness of the Jing we are born into. When I worked with people with developmental disabilities, and many of them were very severe, I occasionally reflected on the poor quality of the Jing they inherited. This is also why you hear in the Qigong community the importance of protecting one's Jing through lifestyle choices. When it's gone, you die.

Qi
Qi is life force, life energy, or often referred to as energy of the universe. It is the flow of life force moving through our bodies that influences our whole well-being. And it is more. Some of my past Qigong

teachers said that Qi is universe intelligence. An intelligence that knows our body and mind so well that if not obstructed will yield "health."

Shen
Shen is our spirit or higher consciousness. Shen has the great potential to communicate with the Dao or the realm of Pure Consciousness. On the lower aspects of the Shen, if there are severe weaknesses of the Shen, our mental faculties could be damaged to the point of mental illness.

Next, we will look at what Master Wu Jyh Cherng says about Jing, Qi, and Shen.

According to Master Wu Jyh Cherng, Jing, Qi, and Shen have many of the same features as already stated. Master Wu Jyh Cherng seems to prefer a simpler way of referring to them. He calls them Essence or Jing, Breath or vital energy, and Spirit or Shen. Shen is active consciousness, which is the force driving the mind. The Qi gives life to both the physical body and the mind-consciousness. There is a fourth important concept, which is Xing, or Nature. This feature is sometimes referred to as Breath or Pure Consciousness.

The uniting of Shen and Qi is a prime goal of Qigong, Taiji, and meditation cultivation. This is the path of duality to non-duality. This is Oneness and happens when the Shen and the Qi fuse. The Xing/Nature precedes the fusion of Shen and Qi because it precedes the separation of these two. Xing originates in Anterior Heaven, thus no differentiation, being equal to Emptiness. Thus Xing is our Absolute True Nature. In our human existence, we have varying degrees of consciousness or energy, and when we develop enough on this path, we may eventually return or recover to the level of Xing/True Nature.

Continued Three Treasures

This next section on the topic of the Three Treasures of Jing, Qi, and Shen is the most complex. In the history and practice of Qigong and Daoist cultivation, there are different views on theory, methodology, and even outcome. My understanding from studying ancient Daoist texts brings me to the realization that there is a practice-oriented way to return Post-Heaven Jing, Qi, and Shen to original Pre-Heaven Jing, Qi, and Shen.

Daoists refer to this way of returning to original nature (Pre-Heaven Jing, Qi, and Shen) as working with the mind and energies in a state of Wu Wei. I wrote in my Qigong and Daoist journals the lessons I learned from Master Meng Zhiling (the Vice-President of the China Daoist Association) during training I did with him in 2016. (See *A Daoist Grows In The Heart*, page 265 and 412) He spoke about Wu Wei and You Wei. He presented Wu Wei as the way of doing things in the most natural and easiest of ways? Keep it simple, he seemed to be saying.

So, in keeping with the principle of Wu Wei, working with Jing, Qi, and Shen is all centered on our abilities to cultivate and maintain an inner state of stillness. It's not the You Wei method of effort and control to move the Qi through the meridians or the feeling of building up of energy or turning the Dantians around like pinwheels. And it's certainly not about building up sexual energies, conjoining with others and falsely thinking you are doing something spiritual. It is about cultivating one's mind to keep it focused on clarity and stillness. To not being so easily distracted by the senses, emotions, and desires of the body and mind. When we practice our Zuowang meditation, we are indeed, doing the inner work of transforming the Jing, Qi, and Shen. I said previously that the Qi has an intelligence of its own, and it applies to not only physical healing but also spiritual healing. Isn't this the transformation of the Three Treasures?

Here's a summary of what I believe are the key ingredients for transforming the Three Treasures back to their original natures. Keep the mind clear and calm, in both times of meditation, and when living in the world. Practice healthy living by eating vibrant foods, exercising often, getting daily rest through sleep, being moderate in your desires, that is, everything from sex to material possessions and ambitions. Avoid attachments, especially to your strong emotions, like anger. And again, our greatest tool for health, longevity, immortality is the degree to which we plunge into the depths of stillness. That's it! That's all we have to do to cultivate the Three Treasures.

The Three Dantians

The Three Dantians are considered to be reservoirs of Qi. There is the Lower Dantian, the Middle Dantian, and the Upper Dantian. There is a general disagreement on the location of the three Dantians. The following is the understanding that makes the most sense to me.

The Lower Dantian is in the lower abdomen. It occupies the space from the navel level across to the Mingmen on the back, and down to the base of the trunk. This is the Dantian generally emphasized in Qigong practice. It is the root of
the tree of life. The Lower Dantian is associated with sexuality, it stores Qi and Jing.

The Middle Dantian is at the level of the heart. It occupies the space from above the Lower Dantian to the base of the neck and throat. It stores the Qi and is related to respiration and the health of the internal organs. It is also known as the heart-mind and it is where yin and yang merge.

The Upper Dantian occupies the head. It holds the Shen, the energy of consciousness, and is related to the brain.

Wei Qi

It seems there is some disagreement about the nature of Wei Qi and which organ systems regulate or control it, or which organ systems strengthen the Wei Qi. But first, a simple definition of what is the Chinese Medicine concept of Wei Qi.

Wei Qi is a protective shield or field of energy that protects both the internal and external body. Most attention is given to the external protective level. This protection is compared to the western medical notion of the immune system.

In Qigong practice, the practitioner intends to increase the strength of the Wei Qi similarly as when they strengthen, stimulate, and cleanse the 12 meridians and extraordinary vessels. The question then arises which meridian should the practitioner focus on to increase the strength of the Wei Qi. I've been exploring a few different explanations of the Wei Qi and here are some of my findings:

> Wei Qi is a classification of Qi that is otherwise known as our protective Qi. It is our first line of defense against external factors that cause illness. ... In traditional Chinese medicine (TCM), our protective Qi is controlled by our lung, a delicate organ susceptible to invasion of the exogenous wind pathogen.

The above is the most basic description of the Wei Qi. The interesting thing to note is the claim that it is the lung energy that controls the Wei Qi. That is the common claim, but not always the case. I'll give another example of a similar point of view but with more detail. The below description is by an acupuncturist and probably represents the most common and acceptable understanding of the Wei Qi.

Morris, Christina. 2020. "The Immune System "Wei Qi." Element, Natural Healing Arts. Elementhealing.com

> In TCM, the external immune system is superficial defense energy called "Wei Qi". Wei Qi is like a shield that surrounds the body, located in the layers of the muscle and skin. This energy controls the opening and the closing of the pores. Wei qi is nourished by the air that we breathe and the foods that we eat. Air quality and diet can directly affect our protective energy. The circulation and

activation of Wei Qi are propelled by the energy of the lungs. Poor lung energy can lead to a poor defense against external pathogens and environmental factors such as wind, cold, heat, dampness, or dryness. Since Wei Qi is controlled by the lungs which are part of the respiratory system, the nasal passage, throat, mucous membranes, and sinuses are commonly affected by an external invasion of pathogens.

But then, I came across a different understanding of Wei Qi that presents a contrary view on Wei Qi. The author is not only a Chinese Medicine doctor but also has a background in the Daoist textual literature of ancient Chinese Medicine.

Yong Ping Jiang, DOM, Ph.D. 2003. "Understanding Wei Qi." March 2003. Vol. 4, Issue 3. Acupuncture Today. Acupuncturetoday.com

> This relationship between the spleen and Wei Qi is highlighted in Chapter 36 of the Ling Shu, which describes the role of each of the five zang (organs) as follows:
> "Among the five zang and six fu, the heart is the sovereign...the lung is the prime minister, the liver is in charge of planning, the spleen is in charge of defending (Wei), the kidney is in charge of supporting."

This passage designates the spleen, not the lung, as the ruler of defense. Nowhere in the Nei Jing does it state that Wei Qi is formed in the lung or originates in the lung. So why do so many modern texts emphasize the lung when talking about Wei Qi? Presumably, it is because the lung and Wei Qi are both said to control the surface of the body.

Indeed, a case can be made that the diffusing function of the lung assists the spread of Wei Qi. But while the lung may help to spread it, the true genesis of Wei Qi lies in the middle burner, and it is here that the healer must focus if he or she is trying to affect this substance. If we ignore the middle burner, we could end up with ineffective therapy when treating Wei Qi deficiency.

I am aware that some modern authors claim that kidney yang is the root source of Wei Qi. This seems to be the result of a misreading of chapter 76 of the Ling Shu. This chapter states that the Wei Qi emerges from the eyes at sunrise and enters the urinary bladder channel, from which it flows successively through the remaining yang channels the rest of the day. At sunset it enters the kidney channel, traveling successively through the remaining yin channels during the night. Both the urinary bladder and kidneys belong to the lower burner, so the lower burner is, in a sense, a starting point for Wei Qi circulation. There is nothing in this chapter, however, that would suggest that Wei Qi is formed in the lower burner; the text is exclusively devoted to a description of circulation.

So, if you want to tonify Wei Qi, you have to focus on the middle burner, especially the spleen. If you bring the lung into the treatment, it will only be to assist the spreading of Wei Qi or to treat concurrent lung symptoms. Kidney yang does not play a direct role in the production of Wei qi, and tonifying kidney yang is only justified if there are clear signs of kidney yang deficiency, such as back and knee pain, cold limbs, etc. Even in these cases, the spleen would have to be tonified as well.

The Qigong State

The Qigong State is an essential component of the practice of Qigong. I often say to my local Qigong students that if one alignment or adjustment of the Qigong State is missing, then you are not doing Qigong. You may still be getting some benefit from exercising but it's not the full Qigong experience. The following section is an extensive explanation of all the components of the Qigong State. Sometimes students or even experienced Qigong practitioners think the Qigong State is a static state that once achieved is then complete. This is absolutely an incorrect way of understanding the Qigong State. You'll see in the information below that the Qigong State keeps evolving as the practitioner deepens their experience of Qigong.

The Three Alignments or Adjustments

The goal of Qigong practice is to attain a state of mind, which is frequently referred to as the Qigong State of Mind. The text, *Chinese Medical Qigong*, calls this state, the state of oneness and involves "bringing the body, breath, and mind into a profound state of oneness." In this summary of the text's explanation on the Three Adjustments, I will highlight its points from the three chapters on body posture, breathing, and mind.

1. Adjustment of Body Posture

Body posture is broken down into stationary or still postures and moving or dynamic body movements.

Stationary or standing posture. The common forms of standing Qigong are included here in this category: Holding the ball in all its variations. Sitting body postures are included here as well, and the purpose of these postures is to assist the person to attain the state of "stillness" required to "reach the Qigong state of oneness."

Dynamic movement practices
There are numerous moving sets, which are done in sequences or individually. An important aspect to mention about dynamic Qigong is its difference from other forms of exercise or general physical training. Qigong training involves the use of the Universal Qi source as its main motivating source. It does not include stiff movements by mechanical force. The Qigong movements are soft and done in a relaxed manner and not stiff or tight as the more general fitness ways of exercising. Some Qigong forms do require firmness and physical strength, for instance, the martial arts forms. For the most part, however, the force of dynamic Qigong comes from the force created by the mind. Any experience of stiffness, fatigue, aches, and numbness in the muscles is usually due to improper use of strength or poor physical condition of the student, rather than the actual Qigong exercise.

2. Adjustment of Breathing

Breathing is directly related to the circulation of internal Qi, and this is key to entering the Qigong State. Common forms of breathing include chest breathing, abdominal, and fetal breathing. Chest breathing is common among people who have developed poor breathing habits. It is to be avoided in Qigong breathing. You know someone is doing chest breathing when you can easily see them lifting their upper chest when they breathe.

Deep abdominal breathing is the most common kind of Qigong breathing. It is also called Dantian or Kidney breathing. This method of breathing focuses on the expanding and contracting of the lower abdominal area. Many people refer to it casually as belly breathing, and quote from the *Daode jing* as "breathing like a baby."

Fetal breathing is what interests me and is key to advanced progression as a Qigong practitioner. In my local Qigong classes, I integrate fetal breathing with abdominal breathing.
Two descriptions of fetal breathing.

A. Imagine the breath entering the navel and exiting from the navel (i.e., the Lower Dantian) thus avoiding a mental focus of breathing from the nose or mouth. Breathe like the baby in the womb, directly through the umbilical cord.
B. Whole-body or just body breathing, or sweat-pores breathing is the other way in which fetal breathing is practiced. The nose or mouth is no longer perceived as the actual passageway for breathing. Practicing body breathing, the Lower

Dantian is the pivot or focus of where the Qi flows from all the pores of the skin, the entire body. With each breath, the whole body breathes, opens, and closes. One of the results of this kind of breathing is the feeling of Qi permeating the whole body and spilling out so one feels unified with the Qi of the universe. This experience greatly contributes to the Qigong State.

3. Adjustment of Mind

Mind adjustment is the process of directing thoughts. This process changes ordinary thinking to enter the Qigong State. In ordinary thinking and living, the mind is usually turned outward and is frequently scattered. In Qigong practice as in most kinds of meditation, the mind is turned inward. The mind guides the Qi inward. This is the leading element of the Three Adjustments. One reaches the Qigong State when the three alignments become integrated into one. The mind adjustments are divided into two kinds:

A. Keep the mind on the body
This means keeping the focus on the body or something else outside of the body, like a tree, an ocean expanse, a mountain, etc. And by the body, it may mean, the Lower Dantian, a particular meridian point, or any area of the body you want to send Qi to. The purpose of keeping the mind on the body is to

filter out distracting, wandering thoughts. This is the original Qigong theory of the mind leads the Qi, or the Qi follows the mind. It is a simple resting of the mind on its focal point. This is close to the Daoist principle of Wu Wei, where the mind settles into the most natural way of doing. If the mind holds rigidly onto the focal point, progress in Qigong is slow and the experience of Qi is minimum or nonexistent.

B. Mental Visualization

This is the process of keeping the mind on imaginary objects, and can also be called observing imagination. The first example, which comes easily to my mind, is Master Wan Sujian's Qigong exercises. In his tonifying of the three Dantians exercise, you tonify each of the three Dantians by imagining Universe Qi flowing into the Dantians. You imagine the vastness of the universe energy flowing into your body. You might use as inspiration the different pictures of the universe that modern science has brought to us through giant telescopes. These images already exist in your memory and imagination. Thus the scope of mental visualization is far wider than that of keeping the mind on the body.

3. Integrating the Three Adjustments Into One

The Three Adjustments are the basic operations in learning and practicing Qigong. When they are all integrated into one, this is the Qigong State. Therefore, integrating them must follow the individual practice of the Three Adjustments. How do you know you have attained Three Adjustments Into One?

Three Adjustments Into One
1. When the Three Adjustments have lost their traces and have merged into one new state. You can hardly tell the difference between each of the individual adjustments.
2. This is the important characteristic of attaining this state of three into one. Initially, one is aware of the integration, one knows one is in the Qigong State. However, having this awareness is an indication that the real "oneness" is still some steps away because the boundary between object and subject is somehow distinguishable in the mind. With more practice and learning, this awareness or "knowing" will also be merged into the integration of the Three Adjustments. Eventually, the state of real oneness will be formed.

The Qigong State is one of gradual development, and best seen as a natural process (Wu Wei), which occurs without the use of willpower or much striving. There is no endpoint, just as in meditation, it is always advancing and evolving.

Advanced Qigong State

The Qigong State has no end and continues to develop as the practitioner masters the skills of Qigong. In this next section, we will explore the advanced Qigong States using the continued guidance from Tianjun Liu O.M.D, the co-author of *Chinese Medical Qigong*. We will use his newer book, *The Key to the Qigong Meditation State: Rujing and Still Qigong*. This English version was originally published in Chinese in the 1990s.

> The final state of Rujing is Ultimate Emptiness, where nothing exists. This is the goal of Rujing when self-awareness will no longer exist. (Liu 2017, 61)

Body Breathing versus Dantian Breathing

In the current literature on Qigong or Daoist breathing, there is a huge focus on breathing in the Lower Dantian. I have nothing against that as it is also part of my practice and even something I encourage my Qigong students to do. But that is not the end of breathing, and there is so little written about the next stages of deeper breathing. Here are some quotes from this book on whole-body breathing:

> When breathing from the Dantian initially switches to body breathing, the Dantian

> breathing point still exists. The breathing channel is not via the mouth and nose. The breath directly gathers and spreads out through the pores of the whole body to the Dantian. Later, the Dantian breathing point will gradually diminish and finally vanish. Breathing in and out of the pores of the whole body will no longer focus on and spread out from the Dantian, but will be soft and continuous and spread evenly through the whole body. (Liu 2017, 262)

This process of breathing becomes more and more subtle until even the rhythm of breathing discontinues and there is only Qi of the body merging with the Qi of the universe. At that point in the process, there is no awareness of the separate body and one attains the state of breathing as the universe.

Ultimate Emptiness

In *The Key to the Qigong Meditation State,* the author says, "Ultimate Emptiness, where nothing exists" is the goal of Qigong practice. (Liu 2017, 61) And how does one arrive at this state of emptiness? Liu states that to attain this state of emptiness, one must begin a process "to forget the existence of your body." Then, after that achievement, "the space on which the body is based will also be forgotten" (2017, 61). Liu says, "When you feel nothing exists, then you are far beyond time and space. 'Emptiness' is everything. It transcends everything" (2017, 62).

Floating and Dissolving Phases into Emptiness

At the end of Liu's book, he gives a guided meditation on how to progress on the path towards emptiness. He presents two concepts of floating and diffusing. The purpose of the floating phase is for the body and heart-mind to become one. While performing a simple Qigong exercise like stationary standing, or even a gentle up and down movement of the arms, like in the Crane Frolic, the body begins a process of feeling more and more weightless. The mind relaxes completely, and you even feel very happy and at ease. While performing your simple Qigong form, or maybe just sitting meditation, you focus on breathing through the pores of the skin. The whole body is breathing. When I practice this, I emphasize the Qi entering my body up from the earth through the soles of my feet, and at the same time heaven Qi descending through the top of my head. I also imagine the Qi entering the rest of my body through all the surface areas. The Qi then eventually makes its way to the Lower Dantian.
The next stage is to forget the focus on the Lower Dantian. As your sense of the body becomes more and more weightless and you have a greater sense of the whole body breathing, no longer will you rely on the Lower Dantian as the place of ultimate breathing.

The flow of breath or Qi will be experienced evenly throughout the whole body. (2017, 262)

There is more to this process according to Liu. The important thing to understand is that this process of floating and diffusing keeps on refining itself again and again until all remnants of self, body, and the material world are completely forgotten. Liu also points out that the posture of the body becomes more critical the further one progresses. This is why he recommends very simple standing postures, which are eventually replaced by either a meditative sitting posture or even lying down. Here's a quote where he describes this:

> Therefore, the operation of body adjustment must match the operation of mind and breathing adjustments. (2017, 264)

Sitting as the best posture for Qigong State

You cannot transcend the physical sensation of body and breathing as long as you are exerting some effort to maintaining a standing posture and an awareness of the physical space around you. He does point out that the sitting cross-legged posture is the best posture to experience these advanced realms of the Qigong State. My experience is that any sitting posture, in a chair or cross-legged on the floor is preferable over lying down, as lying down allows the person to fall asleep too easily.

And that is the full story of the Qigong State. It is far beyond a meditative state where you may feel relaxed and peaceful. The Qigong State is equivalent to our original innate state of Stillness and alignment with the Dao.

Part 5

Chapter 7: Daoist Meditation

You cannot go deep into Qigong unless you have a regular meditation practice. I say this for the benefit of those new to Qigong as well as those who have practiced Qigong for a lengthy time. The method of Daoist meditation that I have practiced for a long time is called Zuowang. It is translated as "sitting and forgetting," or "sitting in oblivion." The unique thing about this method of meditation is that it can be practiced by anyone, regardless of their religious or spiritual preferences. The method is so basic that many traditions have adopted some of its principles and techniques.

In my journal books, I have written extensively about its history, methods, and practices. Zuowang is closely associated with one key Daoist scripture, but don't let that scare you away. It is indeed, a meditation method for all. The scripture is called, the *Zuowang lun,* and translated like I already said, sitting and forgetting.

In my Journal 2, I compared Zuowang meditation to a Catholic contemplative tradition called apophatic prayer or meditation. One of its key texts is called *The*

Cloud Of Unknowing. This book has a double meaning for the aspiring mystic. You enter the cloud of unknowing through the cloud of forgetting. And that is the reason, I sometimes say to my Daoist students, throw all your distracting and wandering thoughts into the cloud of forgetting.

To give you a fuller picture of Zuowang meditation, I will provide you with extensive references from my latest book, *A Daoist Grows In The Heart: Journals Of A Modern-Day Western Daoist Priest*.

I have heard my old teacher explain: Sitting in oblivion is the foundation of long life. Thus we engage perfection to refine the body-form, and once it is pure we merge it into Qi. We retain Dao to refine Qi, and once it is clear we merge it with spirit. The physical structure unified with Dao: this is "attaining Dao." As Dao is without ultimate, how could the immortal ever die? (Kohn 2010, 159)

This above quote from the collection of Daoist scriptures known as the *Zuowang lun* is perhaps the essence of the internal alchemical approach that I follow, and also encourage others. This is the way of tranquility meditation or Zuowang meditation. By "sitting in oblivion" (2010, 159) the adept is going profoundly deep into the internal process of refining Jing, Qi, and Shen, and at such levels, even the concept of the Three Treasures is lost in oblivion and the only goal remaining, the only attainment is that of merging with the Dao. And, are there physical benefits from this attainment? And are there physical benefits even if one does not achieve the complete union with Dao? Well, since the Dao is eternal, "without ultimate" and the scripture says if one practices meditation one will achieve long life and immortality, that sounds like complete health will be within one's grasp. And I would add, that even if one does not make the final attainment, the physical benefits that would accompany the inner transformation of qi to spirit would still be fairly significant, meaning deeply healing.

……….

Put my wandering thoughts into the cloud of forgetting.
Like in the ancient Daoist Chuang Tzu, forget you have a body and forget everything else as well.
The work of Zuowang is to forget the ego, the self, and the personality.
Breathe in ... Not.   Breathe out ... Two
You've cracked open the matrix, broken through the illusions of reality that have kept you separate from everything in the universe.
On the outside door of the matrix is the world of duality.
The other side of the matrix where there is no door is the world of non-duality.

This is things as they are. This is how the Dao sees things, as a state of oneness. But the wonder of it is that from this oneness, one can see the duality of everything as well. This is the depth of the Dao and the Daoist sage.

………..

In my experience, Zuowang is a state of mind expressive of the nondual nature of things whereby the boundaries of separation are dissolved and all things exist simultaneously as empty and full. This is the state of Qigong where we are not separate from the infinite source of Qi pervading all things.

……….

Certainly, this reminds me of our Daoist meditation practice of Zuowang, or what is frequently called sitting and forgetting. The separateness of personal identity is dissolved away through the process of forgetting, and one comes to the insight or awakening of being intimately linked to the totality of the universe. I also refer to this as the experience of Not Two. There are not two things in the entire universe, not even the identity of the circle walker, or the circle, but only the act or event of just walking.

………….

Zuowang is classified as a form of apophatic meditation, which is characterized as not relying on concepts, form, visualization, or any other faculty of the mind. You could call it a mindless way of meditating since it is not of the mind. I like that it keeps reminding you that the practice is to go beyond the mind. However, not tonight, as my mind is full of teapots and tea burners. I am reminded of something I read last year. I included it in my first book. "Why ever think?" This points to the ever-present thinking ego-mind and its false need to be heard.

………..

I have modified my approach to Zuowang meditation based on my readings from the book, *Daoist Meditation*. The added emphasis of placing more focus on the awareness of breathing and the connection to mind or consciousness turns out to have significant consequences. The author, Master Wu Jyh Cherng, calls his method of meditation: Xin Zhai Fa. He says it can be translated as "Purification of the Heart Method or Purification of the Mind Method." and he says, it "promotes purification by emptying the mind of excess thoughts and feelings" (Cherng 2015, 33). Master Wu Jyh Cherng adds that the only requirement for preparing for this practice is to "observe two basic precepts of the Xin Zhai Fa: to sit in silence, preferably in the lotus position, and to concentrate the mind on the air that one breathes" (2015, 34).

....

Before settling into a deep meditative state, a few thoughts passed through my mind. I reflected on my two favorite scriptures, the *Qingjing jing*, and the *Zuowang lun*. These texts contain the essentials of the Daoist path, the attainment of clarity and stillness, the emptiness of self, body and all things, the freedom from desires, the way of forgetting, and the ultimate state of alignment or returning to the Dao. Naturally, as these thoughts passed through my consciousness, I put them one by one into the cloud of forgetting. It doesn't do one any good to have lofty thoughts while one is trying to rest in the state of "constant clarity and stillness." Everything must be forgotten as one breathes in and out, leaving nothing to cling to. Eventually, you must give up the clinging to emptiness and clarity/stillness, as even these things are concepts, thus obstacles. Only rest in the breath and the spirit.

....

A couple of times, the translator used the word, forgetting, to explain what Master Meng was saying. It then dawned on me that he was giving us a lesson on Zuowang meditation, Zuowang, the meditative practice of sitting and forgetting. What he did next was mind-blowing for me. After thoroughly explaining that we need to withdraw from all sensory experiences while meditating, he asked us to prepare for a short session of meditation. He said we would only meditate for 15 seconds. Yes, only 15 seconds. Forget, withdraw from all the senses, and think nothing. Master Meng held his wristwatch in his hands, and said, start! 15 seconds later, he tapped his hands lightly together to indicate to stop. He asked us how we did. I think we were all in a little state of shock. He expected us to totally withdraw from all sensory stimulation. I raised my hand and said I was doing pretty well until I heard the sound of a bird outside. Master Meng, did it again, saying, "try harder." Oh, my god, I said to myself, that is pure Zuowang, that is the state of "Fixation" that Master Wu Jyh Cherng mentions so intensely in his book on Daoist meditation. Here's a quote from *Daoist Meditation* on the general method of Zuowang meditation. See how it is saying the same thing that Master Meng said about turning the senses and the external world inward:

He who meditates finds inner silence… reach…systematic forgetting. This entails the gradual forgetting of external noises, of one's bodily noises and one's words, inner dialogues, and ego… one forgets one's identity, and even that one is sat down, meditating. (2015, 24)

The only difference I see now in these two explanations on this process of meditation is that the emphasis is on experiencing this inner state of "think nothing" in a gradual way versus suddenly, as in a few seconds. I believe, however, that both ways eventually merge as one way. Master Meng did say that when you meditate for longer periods, it becomes more difficult to experience the absence of the senses. I guess the important thing to remember is that in the state of "Fixation" everything is completely forgotten, senses included until you open to the formless realm of Hundun or Anterior Heaven.

………..

As I prepare for my upcoming retreat in April, I am looking at any possible additions to my Zuowang practice. One place that is adding to my understanding of the Zuowang tradition is what I have been discovering in the book by Tianjun Liu, *The Key to the Qigong Meditation State.* In this book, it is clearly stated that the goal of the Qigong State is to end in "Ultimate Emptiness, where nothing exists. (Liu 2017, 61) This is the same goal that is presented in any literature on Zuowang meditation or the Daoist scripture, the *Zuowang lun.* And how does one arrive at this state of emptiness? Liu states that to lose one's ego, which keeps you attached to the body and the material world, one must begin a process "to forget the existence of your body." Then, after that achievement, "the space on which the body is based will also be forgotten" (Liu 2017, 61). These points may not seem that different than traditional sayings on Zuowang, but I believe they lead the practitioner to grow in detachment to not only the ego but also to the world of space and time where the ego functions. Liu says, "When you feel nothing exists, then you are far beyond time and space. 'Emptiness' is everything. It transcends everything" (2017, 62).

I've reported previously in my journal writings that sometimes when I am in a Qigong class or a meditation class that I get fully emerged in a deep meditative state. Then when I come out of it and open my eyes, I am surprised to see that I wasn't alone but teaching a class. I'm not trying to show off by saying that, but I am using myself as an example of "this stuff works."

………..

Thus we are told that by sitting still and utterly calming and clearing the mind, without making any conscious effort to enter any state of meditative trance, you naturally enter into a trance of the most profound kind, wherein the Dao enters the empty space in the mind and causes it to give rise to wisdom. (Eskildsen 2015, 221)

………..

In Zuowang meditation the intention is to align your mind with breathing. The breathing is associated with your inner stillness or your true nature. The main obstacle to this process is all the distractions, which pop up in your mind while you are trying to sit quietly in meditation. I don't have anything new to add to this process. The key is that you just have to practice it. There is no way of getting around that fact.

....

The method of meditation that we will practice on our retreat is known as Zuowang (sitting and forgetting) meditation. Zuowang falls into the passive tradition of meditation to develop serenity, that is, a clear mind, free of any thoughts, and calm from distracting emotions. It aims to allow the wonders of the spiritual world to naturally arise.

....

The Scripture of the *Zuowang lun: Dingguan jing*
He who wishes to attain the Path and reach the Truth must first eliminate all attitudes of perversion and falseness. For there to be no interference in the mind, he must be entirely cut off from external activities and then, sitting in an upright position, inwardly contemplate the 'sense of rectitude'. Each thought that emerges should be swiftly eliminated, and each thought that rises should be immediately controlled, ensuring that one becomes still. Next, ... any chaotic

thoughts and reveries must be eliminated …
(Rinaldini, 2018, 37)

…………

This first instruction seems familiar to us Zuowang practitioners. Sit quietly, turn all your senses inwardly, and be with the breath. Be open to the possibility that sometimes you may be in such a place of stillness that you barely breathe.

Part 6

Chapter 8: The Future Of Qigong: Chong Mai Qigong

The newest area of Qigong that I have been exploring involves the integration of a few simple Qigong movements like, Swimming Dragon, the Crane Frolic, a modified version of Dragon Chases The Pearl, and several others with The Chong Mai Extraordinary Vessel. Most of the exercises have been explained and illustrated in this book. The following discussion will thoroughly explain how all of this goes together. My suggestion is that once you master the exercises and theory presented in this book, you come back to this chapter. Consider it a bonus, along with the chapter on Zuowang meditation. In Qigong, if you apply yourself earnestly and with constancy, you can make great progress. I encourage students to set their goals for the highest attainments. This Chong Mai Qigong will help you attain these lofty goals.

Like my chapter on Zuowang, this material comes from the same book, *A Daoist Grows In The Heart*.

The Chong Mai Qigong set is a new form that I created in 2016 but has continued to evolve into 2017, and may not even be fully realized, as of May 2017.

These notes are taken from my Book 2, and my Book 3.

………..

I have finally come to my last point. And thankfully so, as this last point takes me out of this discourse on the history of Daoism and Longmen lineage and brings us back to the practice of Qigong and circle walking.

In Professor Esposito's explanations on the subsects of the Longmen, she opens up a discussion on the Meridians and the Eight Extraordinary Vessels. She mentions a doctrine, which describes the three Extraordinary Vessels of the Governing, the Conception, and the Thrusting vessels (Chong Mai).

And according to this ancient doctrine, "One can in a flash realize the genuine principle of inner alchemy" (Esposito 2014, 174).

Thus, through certain practices, involving the Governing, the Conception, and the Thrushing Vessels, these energetic vessels are opened and transformed, providing the opportunity for immortality to arise. Professor Esposito quotes the source: "For that reason, it is officially labeled 'the path of the immortals'"(2014, 176). I am leaving out some of the discussion here; it even touches on the topic of Anterior Heaven, one of my favorite Daoist concepts.

………..

I would like to get back to my April 24, 2016 entry from Professor Esposito's book, *Facets of Qing Daoism*. Remember, I said her last point referenced a direct connection to the Eight Extraordinary Vessels and Anterior Heaven, which connects to our circle walking practice. Here's a final quote from her book regarding the Thrushing (Chong Mai) vessel:

The yellow is the Yellow Center (Chong Mai) whose path lies in a middle fissure between the red (Conception Vessel) and the black (Governing Vessel) paths. It is located behind the heart and in front of the spine. If virtue governs the two pnuemas (qi) of the heart and the kidneys, it becomes the central master of the opening and closing.

That which follows this trajectory [i.e. Jing and Qi] temporarily stops in the state of utter emptiness and tranquility because it belongs to the state before Heaven (Xiantian). The realization of an immortal... is dependent on that state. Although one speaks of three different [channels], in reality, they are one. For that reason, it is officially labeled "the path of the immortals" (xiandao). (Esposito 2014, 176)

………..

The Thrusting vessel, also called the Chong Mai vessel, the Thoroughfare vessel, and the Penetrating vessel is located between the Governing and the Conception vessels. This vessel is of such importance for our Qigong and Daoist cultivation that I cannot overstate its value. Any book I pick up on the Eight Extraordinary Vessels gives it supreme ratings. It is said that the Chong Mai vessel "mirrors the energetic properties of the unfolding of the Tao" (Twicken 2013, 46). Furthermore, it is said that the Chong Mai vessel "creates all channels, and it can influence all of them" (Twicken 2013, 46). Considering these spiritual and energetic aspects of the Chong Mai vessel we can understand why Tom Bisio, in his circle walking book, places great emphasis on the Pushing the Palms Down posture:

The Downward Sinking Palm is the first palm that you practice because the position of the arms and body particularly stimulates and opens Du Mai, Ren Mai, and Chong Mai. When these channels are activated and opened, it is easier to open the other Meridians and channels. (Bisio 2012, 176)

....

Perhaps the energetic portal to the state of Anterior Heaven is through the Chong Mai vessel. In our Zuowang practices, there is a strong connection between breath awareness and the Lower Dantian. And the more we sink our awareness into the depths of the Lower Dantian through stillness and clarity, the more we open and pass through the portal of the Chong Mai. Thus, walking in a circle in the Pushing The Palms Down posture is an ally to Zuowang practice to open the Chong Mai and emerge out the other side in the realm of Anterior Heaven. Wow.

....

I just finished a short session of Pushing The Palms Down. One aspect of this posture to keep in mind is a feeling of pushing the Qi down the front of the body and allowing the Qi to flow up the back. You can encourage this up and down flow of Qi by simply uniting it to the breath. Exhale, follow the Qi/breath down the front, inhale follow the Qi/breath up the back. The rest of the body should be relaxed with a feeling of sinking into the earth. You can go further in connecting with the Chong Mai by narrowing your Qi/breath to simply move up and down this channel in a single column. Allow yourself to dissolve away in your Qigong state. Forget the circle, and forget the image of energy moving up and down the body. Forget the body, and forget the person doing all this. Walking, breathing, not thinking. The birds singing.

....

In last Wednesday's Qigong class, one of my long-term students and I created a new Qigong set based on the Chong Mai channel and the Governing and Conception channels. I presented some guidelines to help narrow down the selection of which particular Qigong movements would best support these extraordinary channels. We came up with six Qigong exercises taken from my complete list of exercises. I explained to Tracy, my student, that even though I presented some guidelines in the selection process, there is not any actual right and wrong choice for what we did. My point is we just made some choices based on simple Qigong principles.

We started the practice with Swimming Dragon and emphasized standing straight and pivoting and turning and twisting side to side. We imagined Qi moving up and down the Chong Mai channel, as well as up and down the back and front channels.
We next transitioned to a modified form of Dragon Chases The Pearl and focused on the Qi moving up and down these same channels as in the first step. In my version of Primordial Wuji Qigong, there is a middle phase of circulating the hands up and down in front of the lower Dantian. This was the third step.

Qi moving along the pathway of these channels, top to bottom again and again. Then came the wings of arms rising and falling of the Crane Frolic. We stretched up and sank as the Qi followed its course. After this flapping of the wings, we slowly moved into the Compassionate Buddha Qigong.

The movements allowed a complete letting go of any residual tension or stress.

Double Hands Hold Up The Heavens is the last exercise to emphasize the Qi moving along the Chong Mai channel. The set closes with an extended gathering of the three breaths to the feet, the legs and the upper body.

My personal experience with this set was very powerful. It created in me a deep Qigong state of mind. And on a deeper level, I can see the potential for passing through the portal to the Anterior Heaven state of being and feeding directly off of the Pre-Celestial Qi of the Universe.

………..

The major sequence is the set of six exercises that stimulate the flow of Qi up and down the three central pathways of the Governing (Du), Conception (Ren), and Chong Mai vessels.

The Qigong exercises are Swimming Dragon, Dragon Chases The Pearl, Phase Two of Primordial Wuji Qigong, Crane Frolic, Compassionate Buddha Qigong, and the Double Hands Hold Up The Heavens.

…………

The breathing pattern for the major sequence (set of 6 movements) is sometimes difficult. I am leaving room for flexibility here for practitioners to find their breathing patterns. My method of breathing is to align the inhaling with a sense of mind/energy descending to the base of the Chong Mai vessel, and then exhaling as the mind-energy rises to the Baihui top of the head.

Part 7

Chapter 9: The Conclusion

For a conclusion to this book, I decided to end it with one of my most powerful forms of Qigong, Compassionate Buddha Qigong. It is an original form that I created 20 years ago, and it is still relevant today, and probably, essential for the world health crisis we are in. Enjoy, Be Silent, Heal Yourself, Heal The World.

The following description of Compassionate Buddha Qigong is taken from my Qigong Certification training manual.

Compassionate Buddha Qigong

Compassionate Buddha Qigong is a form of Qigong that came to me intuitively one late summer evening back in September of 1999. I had decided to go for a walk in my neighborhood in Sebastopol. I remember being filled with energy and walking for the sake of just walking. I was saying my Tibetan mantra- Om Mani Peme Hung. Eventually, I found myself at a local park. The time was approximately 7 pm, and so there was still plenty of daylight.

After walking for about a half-hour, I was ready for some stationary activity. I noticed several trees clustered together and forming something of a grove with an open area for me to do some Qigong. Finding my spot, I just stood in an upright position. I remember thinking of how readily I usually move into one of the Standing Qigong positions with raised arms. This time, however, I stood with arms relaxed at my sides, and feet firmly planted on the ground and having no expectations of 'what next.' I intended to simply stand there and experience all the energy around me. I felt a great aliveness and a wanting to expand more and more into this feeling of emptiness. My body seemed to be holding me back from fully letting go. It felt like a heavy burden. Instinctively, I began to move my hands. First, my hands moved to the front of my body, fingers pointing at each other, palms turned upwards, slowly lifting them, as if lifting an object. Raising my hands to my face level, and then turning my palms outward, and lifting further to above my head until my arms were fully extended. Continuing this movement to the sides, making a full circle and lowering my hands until they were in the same starting position in front of my body.

At first, I just kept repeating this basic pattern. As I continued, I began to slightly bend my knees as if reaching deep into the earth. My mind moved further into the space surrounding me. I felt in complete harmony with the earth, the trees, everything around me, including the sky and beyond. It then occurred to me that it was more than just energy, but another aspect of the Qi that I was experiencing. I'll call it the compassionate nature of the universe. I could give it all sorts of names, but it all boils down to the realization that at a fundamental level of reality there is love and compassion throughout existence.

As I progressed in this Qigong state, my movements became slower and slower. I slowed down so much that it felt as if my breathing was regulating my movements by tiny, tiny increments, and sometimes no movements at all. I felt I was doing an extremely slow standing Qigong practice. The positions I held the longest were with my arms outstretched to the sides, hands at waist level. Eventually, I did remain motionless for what seemed like an eternity.

At some point, I began to move again, but very slowly. As my movements increased in pace, I visualized sending out healing rays of Qi and love to all beings. I thought of my family and imagined them engulfed in this healing Qi field. The faces of friends and students came to my mind. It felt like they were there with me, healing from this outpouring of nature's radiance. Gradually, my thoughts turned to all people, all things, including the much-needed healing of our planet, Earth. It was like a veil of darkness or illusion had lifted and it was clear that all things are pure energy and in harmony with the Great Tao, the Great Buddha, and the Great Christ. I looked at the surrounding trees, the people playing in the park, the grass and dirt beneath my feet, and intuitively knew that we were indeed just One Being, and that was good. A great wave of appreciation swept over my body as I completed my movements. I had come up with a new Qigong practice, and I was excited to tell my students about it.

Basic Movements & Guidelines

Compassionate Buddha Qigong (CBQ) consists of circular movements using the arms and hands and bending the legs to move the body up and down.

Mind Visualization
Before you begin any movements, stand with your hands relaxed at your sides. Expand your mind into the Qi field surrounding you. Relax deeply. Visualize that the ground beneath you is dissolving and you are suspended in space. Think of yourself as a cosmic energy body of light. Then begin your movements.

First, I'll explain the arm and hand movements. Start with hands at lower abdominal area, palms turned upwards, and fingertips pointing toward each other. (Figure 35) Slowly raise them in front of the body as if lifting an object. At approximately head level, turn the palms outwards so that the backs of your hands are facing you. Continue moving your hands upwards and outwards in a large circular direction. Your hands and arms move out to the sides (Figure 36-37) and then return to the starting position. (Figure 35) As your hands reach outward, your mind soars into the emptiness of deep space. The more you expand your mind, the more you will experience the release of negative influences and the abundance of health.

Next, we'll look at the up and down movements. To begin with, stand with the feet shoulder-width apart, or slightly more. At the start of the movements (perhaps the first 3-5 up and down movements) bend at the knees as if squatting. (Figure 38) Sometimes you may squat to the floor. If you practice the form correctly, you will gain great stability and strength in the legs. You will also increase the flow of Qi in your body. The rest of the practice will be done in a standing position.

The other basic element of this practice is the speed of moving the arms and hands changes throughout the session. You start at a slow-moderate pace. As you progress, the movements become slower, and eventually, all movement stops completely. The question of whether the eyes should be open or closed is a matter of personal preference. Do what feels comfortable.

The Letting Go Process
The heart of CBQ is the process of letting go and emptying everything from the mind and body. There is no right or wrong way of accomplishing this letting go. For instance, as
you move up and down, breathing in and out, you mentally feel like you are letting go of tensions, stresses, toxins, etc. from your body. Mentally imagine the muscles, the bones, and so on, releasing … As you progress, go deeper into the internal organs. Be creative in where the mind goes to release. And don't forget your emotions, letting go of anger, worry, sadness, etc. This process will vary every time you practice CBQ.

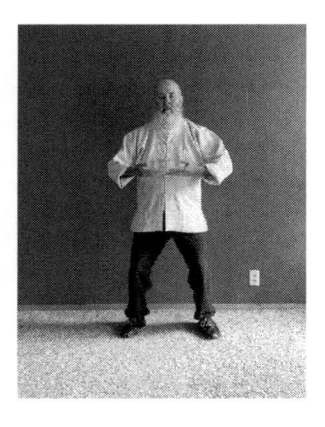

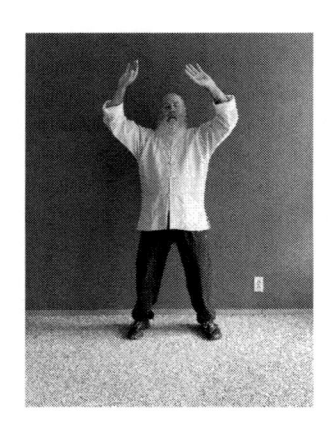

Figure 35   Figure 36

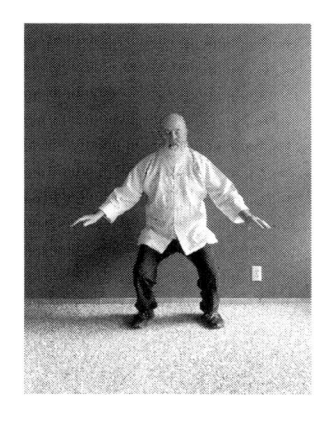

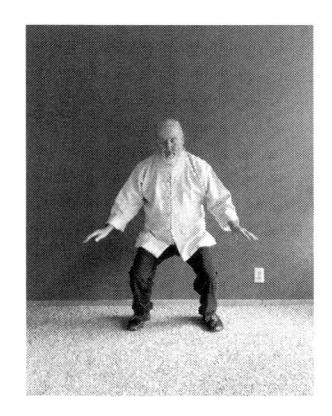

Figure 37   Figure 38

As you go through this process of releasing, your movements are becoming slower and slower, as I said above. When you complete this letting go process, that is the time to be completely still, deep in your Qigong State. While in this deep state of stillness, you are filled with cosmic light and emptiness. Your mind is full of stillness, but your awareness radiates with healing compassion for the world, for all peoples. For the moment, you are the Compassionate Buddha or Compassionate Christ. Coming out of this internal state of quietness and stillness, you move your arms again, you mentally send out compassionate energies to the world, to whomever you wish.

Closing

At the end of a practice session, it is important to gather and store the Qi in the Lower Dantian. This is done by mentally focusing on the Qi flowing into the

Lower Dantian, including the kidneys. Visualize the Qi building up a vast, internal, silent reservoir that is radiating out in compassion to all beings.

Final reflections
It is important to realize that there is a progression of healing that the practitioner moves through. First, there is the purifying phase, then the self-healing phase, and finally the healing of others. I often think of the planet Earth as a living being which needs healing on a deep level.
Again, I say:

Enjoy, Be Silent, Heal Yourself, Heal The World

Bibliography

Bisio, Tom. 2012. *Ba Gua Circle Walking Nei Gong: The Meridian Opening Palms Of Ba Gua Zhang.* Denver, Colorado: Outskirts Press, Inc.

Cohen, Ken. 2020. "In the company of Cranes: Ancient Teachers of Qigong." *Qi, The Journal of Traditional Eastern Health and Fitness.* Spring. Volume 30, No. 1. Temecula, CA: Insight Graphics.

Deadman, Peter. 2016. *Live Well Live Long.* Hove, UK: The Journal of Chinese Medicine Ltd.

Eskildsen, Stephen. 2015. *Daoism, Meditation, and the Wonders of Serenity: From the Latter Han Dynasty (25-220) to the Tang Dynasty (618-907).* New York: State University of New York.

Esposito, Monica. 2014. *Facets of Qing Daoism.* Wil / Paris: UniversityMedia. www.universitymedia.org

Frost, Mark. 2020. "Windscreen Powder (Yu Ping Feng San)." Mayway.com newsletter. April 22, 2020.

Jiang, Yong Ping, DOM, Ph.D. 2003. "Understanding Wei Qi." March 2003. Vol. 4, Issue 3. Acupuncture Today. Acupuncturetoday.com

Kohn, Livia. 2010. *Sitting in Oblivion: The Heart of Daoist Meditation*. Dunedin: Three Pines Press.

Liu, Tianjun. 2017. *The Key to the Qigong Meditation State, Rujing, and Still Qigong*. Philadelphia, PA: Singing Dragon.

Morris, Christina. 2020. "The Immune System "Wei Qi." Element, Natural Healing Arts. Elementhealing.com

Rinaldini, Michael. 2010-2020. *Rites of the American Dragon Gate Lineage*. Collected and Arranged by Michael Rinaldini (Shifu Li Chang Dao). Unpublished Collection.

_____ . 2020. *A Daoist Grows In The Heart: Journals Of A Modern-Day Western Daoist Priest*. Sebastopol, CA: Independently Published.

Twicken, David. 2013. *Eight Extraordinary Channels, Qi Jing Ba Mai*. London: Singing Dragon, Jessica Kingsley Publishers.

Wu Jyh Cherng. 2015. *Daoist Meditation: The Purification of the Heart Method of Meditation and Discourses on Sitting and Forgetting (Zuo Wang Lun) by Sima Cheng Zhen*. London: Singing Dragon.

Yan, Zhen. 2020. "COVID-19: Exercise may protect against deadly complication: May prevent or reduce the severity of acute respiratory distress syndrome." (ARDS) University of Virginia School of Medicine. EurekAlert. Eurekalert.org

About The Author

Shifu Michael Rinaldini (Lichangdao) is the director of the Qigong & Daoist Training Center in Sebastopol, CA, where he teaches classes and leads annual retreats in Qigong, Circle Walking, Daoist meditation, and Chinese Food Therapy. For advanced students, he offers a Qigong Certification program of 200 hours in Qigong and introductory Daoist practices. His program is available locally, nationally, and internationally, having students throughout the USA, Canada, UK, Mexico, Slovak Republic, Austria, Australia, Finland, and elsewhere.

Shifu Michael is also the founder of the American Dragon Gate Lineage, a Daoist non-monastic lineage with a membership of over 25 ordained or priests-in-training. His training is limited to serious students of the Dao who wish to become ordained Daoist priests of the Lineage (ADGL) after three years of practice and study. Students perform the studies at their residences but attend group retreats throughout the 3-year training phase.

For more information on Shifu Michael, and his training, visit his web site: www.qigongdragon.com

Printed in Great Britain
by Amazon